THE LONGEVITY DIET PLAN

Step by Step guide to Lose Weight, Eat Healthy and Feel Better Following this Lifestyle with Tasty Recipes.

By David Clark

BOOK1

BOOK2

INTERMITTENT FASTING

55 Recipes For Intermittent Fasting and Healthy Rapid Weight Loss

By David Clark

Introduction:

Intermittent fasting is an example of eating that alternates between times of fasting, normally devouring just water, and non-fasting, generally eating anything a person needs regardless of how stuffing. In the evening time, a person can eat anything he needs for 24 hours and fast for the following 24 hours. This way to deal with weight control is by all accounts upheld by science, just as strict and social practices throughout the planet. Followers of Intermittent fasting guarantee that this training is an approach to turn out to be more careful about food.

Also, an Intermittent fasting diet is somewhat unique from ordinary fasting. This kind of transient fasting doesn't decrease fat-consuming chemicals. Truth be told, logical exploration has shown that the specific inverse occurs and you will begin expanding the movement of fat-consuming catalysts.

An incredible part of Intermittent fasting is that there isn't a lot of exertion included. You can carry on with life, go out to eat, still have your favorite food sources and a periodic treat. The weight loss can be quick or consistent relying upon how you approach it. You can be as severe or loose about your eating as you need and still get more fit. Eating this way is useful for breaking levels as well.

To benefit from Intermittent fasting, you need to fast for at any rate 16 hours. At 16 hours or more, a portion of the stunning advantages of Intermittent fasting kicks in. A simple method to do this is to just skip breakfast each day. This is in reality extremely solid, however, many people will try to disclose to you in any case. By skipping breakfast, you are permitting your body to go into a caloric shortfall, which will enormously build the measure of fat you can consume and the weight you can lose.

Since your body isn't caught up with processing the food you ate, it has the opportunity to zero in on consuming your fat stores for energy and for purifying and detoxifying your body. If you think that it's hard to skip breakfast, you can rather skip a meal, even though I track down this considerably more troublesome.

It truly doesn't make any difference, yet the objective is to broaden the timeframe you spend fasting and loss the measure of time you spend eating. If you have a meal at 6 PM and don't eat until 10 the following morning, you have refrained for 16 hours. Longer is better, however, you can see some beautiful extraordinary changes from every day 16 hours fast.

Chapter: 1 Breakfast

A better smooth fish pasta heat loaded with heaps of vegetables and surprisingly some mysterious beans. The ideal family-accommodating pasta dish that works for babies and adults. There are alternatives to make this gluten-free, lactose-free, or even dairy-free.

Ingredients:

- 1 block chicken stock
- Salt and pepper
- 4 tbsp. Parmesan cheddar
- 2 tsp lemon juice
- 1.25 cups light coconut milk
- 1.5 tbsp. whole meal flour
- 1 tbsp. margarine
- 1 tsp coconut oil
- 425 g canned fish in spring water
- 1/4 cup whole meal breadcrumbs
- 1 cup frozen or tinned peas or corn or veg of decision

Method:

- Preheat oven to 180C.
- Channel fish and spot in a blending bowl.

- Add corn to the bowl and blend well.
- Season with salt and pepper.
- Cook cubed onions in coconut oil until delicate.
- Add onions to fish blend, mix well.
- Add spread to frypan and soften.
- Pour in coconut milk and gradually add the flour, whisking continually to stay away from knots.
- Add 3 tbsp. of the Parmesan cheddar and the lemon juice.
- Disintegrate the stock shape and sprinkle over the top, then add prepared to taste.
- Blend well.
- Pour sauce over the fish combination and mix until very much consolidated.
- Tip into stove confirmation dishes – it is possible that one huge dish, or personal dishes.
- Combine as one whole meal breadcrumb and the leftover Parmesan cheddar and sprinkle over the fish blend.
- Cook in the oven for 25 minutes and afterward grill for a further 5-10 mins until brilliant earthy colored on top.
- Fill in with no guarantees or with steamed greens, pasta, salad, or rice.

2: Sweet Potato & Black Bean Burrito

Sound Sweet Potato and Black Bean Burrito are loaded down with such a lot of goodness. Your number one tortilla or wrap is loaded up with chime pepper, yam, black beans, avocado, and earthy colored rice for a nutritious dish with stunning flavor. These are normally gluten-free (contingent upon the tortilla) veggie-lover burritos that make an astonishing breakfast, lunch, or dinner that is prepared in less than 30 minutes.

Ingredients:

- fine grain ocean salt
- 1 big red onion, cut
- avocado oil (I utilized Primal Kitchen)
- ground chipotle powder
- 4–6 burrito estimated tortillas
- hot sauce or salsa, whenever wanted (I love a tomatillo one with these!!)
- 1 large or 2 little yams, slashed into 1/2" blocks (no compelling reason to strip, simply wash them well!!)
- 1 15-ounce container of black beans, flushed and depleted

Method:

- Preheat stove to 400 F.
- On a material-lined dish, toss red onions and yams with enough avocado oil to cover and a liberal measure of salt and some chipotle powder.
- Prepare for 20-30 minutes, tossing a couple of times, until yams are effectively penetrated with a fork and onions are earthy colored (whatever's cooking excessively, move more to the middle!).
- Add the black beans to the oven and toss to blend.
- Warm tortillas for 30 seconds on each side to make them flexible (this is too essential to keep them from breaking when you try to overlap them!) then do a line

of the black bean and yam combination down the center.

- Add hot sauce if utilizing. Crease in sides and roll. As far as I might be concerned, this made 5 burritos, yet it'll shift dependent on the size of your tortillas. Wrap burritos in foil, and hold up!
- To plan, microwave, or utilize a toaster to warm when prepared to eat.

3: Pb and J Overnight Oats

These **PB&J Overnight Oats** are a definitive make-ahead breakfast that will keep you powered and empowered throughout the day with whole-grain moved oats, chia seeds, peanut butter, and jam. Make your oats with this natively constructed Chia Seed Jam and add your number one fresh organic product. Overnight cereal is a steady staple in my morning meal routine since it is something I can prepare early and I realize will keep me full throughout the morning.

Ingredients:

- 1 cup moved oats
- 1 tablespoon chia seeds
- 1 cup unsweetened almond milk
- 1/2 tablespoon maple syrup
- 1 tablespoon jam or jelly
- 2 tablespoons rich peanut butter

Method:

- Spot all ingredients short the jam in a glass Tupperware and blend.

- Cover and let sit in the cooler for at any rate 2 hours or overnight.
- In the morning, twirl in some jam and appreciate cold.

4: Porridge with Apple and Cinnamon

Porridge is consistently an extraordinary method to begin the day, regardless of whether you're an infant, youngster, or grown-up. My apple and cinnamon porridge is pressed brimming with flavor. You can eat it also, or jazz it up for certain additional ingredients - I like walnut nuts and poppy seeds. My variant is appropriate for vegetarians; however, you can utilize your preferred milk.

Ingredients:

- 2 tbsp. honey
- 1 section moved oats to 2 sections of milk
- 1 apple
- Touch of salt
- Small bunch toasted walnuts, generally chopped

Method:

- Measure the porridge in a little glass then add it to a little sauce container with twice the milk.
- Spot the pan on medium-high heat and bring to the bubble, then turn off the heat.
- Add a touch of salt and mix reliably until you have a thick, velvety blend, this will take about 8-10minutes.
- Mesh the apple and mix half of it into the porridge, then add the cinnamon and honey and blend well.

- Serve the porridge in a bowl then top it with the remainder of the ground apple, some more cinnamon, and honey.
- Sprinkle the toasted walnuts on top, it's a decent option to add some virus milk over the top if you like.

5: Greek Chickpea Waffles

Waffles are a morning meal staple which is as it should be. They're regularly fleecy, sweet, and covered in margarine—who could want anything more? However, in case you're attempting to go for something somewhat better (and would prefer not to hit your daily calorie quantity just after breakfast), choosing appetizing waffles can make breakfast in a hurry quite a lot more stimulating.

Ingredients:

- 1/2 tsp. heating pop
- 3/4 c. chickpea flour
- 1/2 tsp. salt
- 6 huge eggs
- 3/4 c. plain 2% Greek yogurt
- Cucumbers, parsley, yogurt, tomatoes, scallion, and lemon juice, for serving

Method:

- Heat stove to 200°F. Set a wire rack over a rimmed heating sheet and spot it on the stove. Heat waffle iron per bearings.
- In a big bowl, preparing pop, whisk together flour, and salt.

- In a little bowl, whisk together yogurt and eggs.
- Mix wet ingredients into dry ingredients.
- Gently cover waffle iron with nonstick cooking shower and, in clumps, drop ¼ to ½ cup player into each segment of iron and cook until brilliant earthy colored, 4 to 5 minutes.
- Move to the stove and keep warm. Rehash with the leftover player.
- Serve finished off with cucumbers, tomatoes, and scallion threw with olive oil, pepper, salt, and parsley.
- Shower with yogurt blended in with lemon juice.

6: Avocado Quesadillas

Firm quesadillas loaded up with beans, ringer pepper, sautéed onions, avocado, and bunches of cheddar. These avocado black bean quesadillas are filling and make an extraordinary vegan feast as well. They make an extraordinary breakfast and are very filling as well!

Ingredients:

- 4 delicate flour or corn tortillas
- 1 avocado, hollowed, stripped, and cut into pieces
- 4 ounces Manchego cheddar, cut
- 16 canned or jolted jalapeño cuts

Method:

- Get out 1 tortilla on a work surface.

- Spot about a fourth of the cheddar on one half, not very close to the edge so the cheddar won't soften out as it cooks.
- Top cheddar with a fourth of the avocado and four jalapeño cuts.
- Overlap tortilla fifty-fifty over filling to frame a half-circle.
- Heat a grill container or oven over medium heat.
- Slide uncooked quesadilla onto the oven.
- Crunch down with a weight or simply press momentarily with a spatula.
- Cook 1 moment, then flip the quesadilla and flame broil brief more or until cheddar is liquefied.
- Move the quesadilla to a cutting board and cut it into 6 wedges. Serve right away. Rehash with residual ingredients. Makes 24 wedges.

7: Veggie lover Fried 'Fish' Tacos

This recipe for veggie lover fish tacos is loaded with flavor yet, however, so natural to plan! There's no untidy twofold digging of these children, a too basic one bowl fish 'n chips-style hitter is all you need to get incredibly firm vegetarian "fish" bits ideal for ingredient your Baja fish taco wanting. These veggie-lover fish tacos are stunningly presented with an avocado plate of mixed greens and my blackberry margaritas.

Ingredients:

- 2/3 cup water

- 1/2 cup panko breadcrumbs
- 2 teaspoons nori powder (discretionary, for an 'off-putting' taste)
- 1/2 teaspoon salt
- 2 tablespoons lemon juice
- 1/2 cup flour
- 1 (14 ounces) bundle firm or extra firm tofu, depleted and squeezed
- 2 tablespoons soy sauce or tamari
- 1 tablespoon cornstarch

Rich Lime Slaw:

- 2 tablespoons lime juice
- 1/3 cup veggie-lover mayo of decision
- 1/2 teaspoon stew powder
- 1/4 teaspoon ground cumin
- 1/4 teaspoon salt
- 1/2 teaspoon garlic powder
- 4–5 cups finely destroyed cabbage

Method:

- Preheat the stove to 450 degrees F.
- Make the tofu fish sticks: In one bowl, combine as one the soy sauce, lemon juice, and nori powder.
- In another bowl, whisk together the flour and cornstarch, then gradually race in the water to make a play.
- Put the excess breadcrumbs and salt in a third bowl.

- Cut the tofu into finger-like strips, then plunge into the lemon bowl, the flour player, and finely the panko.
- Spot on a lubed preparing sheet and proceed with the remainder of the tofu.
- Heat for 10 minutes, then flip and cook an extra 8 minutes, or until brilliant earthy colored and fresh.
- While the tofu is cooking, whisk together the elements for the slaw in a big bowl: the mayo, lime squeeze, and preparing.
- Taste, adding more flavors/salt depending on the situation.
- Then include the cabbage and throw well, proceeding to throw the cabbage will cover the cabbage and begin to separate it so it's simpler to eat.
- Warm the tortillas, then partition the tofu onto the tortillas and top with slaw.
- Spurt with all the fresher lime juice, whenever wanted, and appreciate!

8: Peach Berry Smoothie

Smoothies are one of my #1-morning meals or evening jolts of energy (so extraordinary when you live someplace blistering!). I love that there are in a real sense unlimited blends and in its single direction my children will cheerfully eat (drink?) their veggies and pack in some extra organic product. This blueberry peach smoothie dairy-free, normally improved and so delightful on account of delicious peaches and blueberries.

Ingredients:

- 1/2 cup almond milk or most loved juice
- 3/4 cup Driscoll's Blueberries
- 1 Tbsp. ground flaxseeds
- 1/2 cup non-fat plain Greek yogurt
- 2 Tablespoons honey
- 1 little peach, generally slashed, or 1/2 cup frozen peaches
- 3 Ounces ice solid shapes (not required if utilizing frozen peaches)

Method:

- Mix blueberries, peach, almond milk, flaxseeds, honey, yogurt, and ice in a blender until pureed and smooth, mixing a few times.
- Serve right away.

Beginning your day with a sound Green Breakfast Smoothie is an incredible method to get empowered and feel great. This one is sound and delicious … a triumphant combo. Drinking this daily smoothie is the thing that assisted me with getting the body and energy to do some unimaginable things. Most smoothies are made with simply foods grown from the ground, which is high in sugar and can cause aggravation. A green smoothie, then again, is made with fruit, plant-based fluid, and verdant greens.

Ingredients:

- 1 huge mango, frozen
- 1 green apple, cored
- 1/2 English cucumber
- 6 little leaves of romaine (or 3 modest bunches of spinach)
- 1/2 lemon, stripped and cultivated
- 2 celery stems
- cold sifted water to mix (around 2 cups)

Method:

- Spot everything into a fast blender and mix until smooth.
- Serve and appreciate right away.

It's another best recipe for irregular fasting referenced in the morning meal list. You can make it easy and within a short time. It's truly tasty and everybody will like it.

Ingredients:

- 1/2 teaspoon salt
- 1 tablespoon ground lemon strip
- 4 boneless skinless chicken bosom parts
- 5 tablespoons fresh lemon juice, isolated
- 1 teaspoon olive oil, partitioned
- 2 tablespoons olive oil, partitioned
- 1 garlic clove, finely cleaved
- 1/4 teaspoon ground black pepper
- 2 garlic cloves, cooked and pounded
- 1/2 teaspoon ocean salt
- 1 medium tomato, cultivated and finely cleaved
- 1/4 teaspoon fresh ground pepper
- 1/4 cup little green pimento-stuffed olives, meagerly cut
- 2 tablespoons fresh basil leaves, finely cut
- 3 tablespoons escapades, washed
- 1 big avocado, split, hollowed, stripped, and finely cleaved

Method:

- In a sealable plastic pack, consolidate chicken and marinade of the lemon strip, 2 tablespoons lemon juice, garlic, 2 tablespoons olive oil, salt, and pepper.

- Seal sack and refrigerate for 30 minutes.
- In a bowl, whisk together the leftover 3 tablespoons lemon juice, staying 1/2 teaspoons olive oil, ocean salt, simmered garlic, and fresh ground pepper.
- Blend in tomato, green olives, escapades, basil, and avocado; put in a safe spot.
- Eliminate chicken from the sack and dispose of marinade.
- Grill over medium-hot coals for 4 to 5 minutes for every side or to the ideal level of doneness.
- Present with Avocado Tapenade.

11: Meal Club Tilapia Parmesan

This is a very basic dish, so several excessively basic side dishes are all you need. These Sautéed Green Beans with Cherry Tomatoes. I would simply keep it simple. I think one normal misinterpretation of this recipe is that it ought to be fresh. "Crusted" in this case simply implies that it is shrouded in Parmesan.

Ingredients:

- black pepper
- 1 scramble hot pepper sauce
- 2 tablespoons lemon juice
- 2 lbs. tilapia filets
- 1/2 cup ground parmesan cheddar
- 3 tablespoons mayonnaise
- 4 tablespoons margarine, room temperature
- 3 tablespoons finely slashed green onions

- 1/4 teaspoon dried basil
- 1/4 teaspoon preparing salt

Method:

- Preheat oven to 350 degrees.
- In a buttered 13-by-9-inch heating dish or jellyroll container, lay filets in a solitary layer.
- Do not stack filets.
- Brush top with juice.
- In a bowl consolidate cheddar, margarine, mayonnaise, onions, and flavors.
- Blend well in with a fork.
- Prepare fish in preheated oven for 10 to 20 minutes or until fish simply begins to piece.
- Spread with cheddar combination and prepare until brilliant earthy colored, about 5minutes.
- Heating time will rely upon the thickness of the fish you use.
- Watch fish intently with the goal that it doesn't overcook.
- Makes 4 servings.
- Note: This fish can likewise be made in an oven.
- Sear 3 to 4 minutes or until practically done.
- Add cheddar and sear another 2 to 3 minutes or until sautéed.

Broccoli Curry is a simple and sound sauce or curry dish that can be presented with hot phulkas or steamed rice. This lovely green vegetable is a storage facility of nutrients and minerals. This recipe safeguards every one of the first supplements of broccoli since it doesn't overcook the broccoli florets.

Ingredients:

- 1 – Potato
- 1 - Broccoli
- 1 - Onion
- 1/2 tsp - Ginger and Garlic glue
- 1/4 cup - Cut Corn
- 1/2 tsp - Dhania Jeera powder
- 1/2 tsp - Urad dal
- Salt and Red Chili powder to taste
- 1 squeeze - Turmeric powder
- 1/2 tsp - Mustard seeds
- 4 tsp - Oil

Method:

- Cut the broccoli into little pieces and cook in the microwave for 6 minutes.
- Heat oil in a container and add urad dal, mustard seeds and fry them to a brilliant brown tone.
- Cleave the onion and potato into pieces, add it to the above blend and fry till the potato is bubbled.

- Add to the abovementioned, ginger and garlic glue, dhania and jeera powder, a little turmeric powder, and if you need 1/2 tsp garam masala.
- Add the cooked broccoli pieces alongside slicing corn and salt to taste and red stew powder, and cook it for 5 minutes.
- Your broccoli curry is fit to be presented with one or the other rice or chapatti.

13: Pie Maker Zucchini Slice Muffins

Here is another best recipe for your morning meal. You can undoubtedly make this recipe at your home. It's an astonishing recipe that everybody will very much want to have.

Ingredients:

- 200g yam, stripped, coarsely ground
- 80ml (1/3 cup) extra virgin olive oil
- 2 medium zucchini (about 300g), managed, coarsely ground
- 5 eggs, delicately whisked
- 150g (1 cup) self-rising flour
- 100g (1 cup) Perfect Italiano Perfect Bakes cheddar (mozzarella, cheddar, and parmesan)

Method:

- Heat 1 tablespoon of the oil in a medium non-stick oven over medium-high heat.
- Add the yam and cook, mixing periodically, for 5 minutes or until mollified. Move to a big bowl.

- Add the zucchini, flour, cheddar, egg, and remaining oil.
- Season well and mix to join.
- Preheat the pie producer.
- Fill the pie producer openings with a yam blend.
- Close, cook for 8 minutes.
- Rehash with the excess blend.
- Serve warm or cold.

14: Simmered Broccoli with Lemon-Garlic and Toasted Pine Nuts

So natural thus great. Simmered broccoli with lemon zing, pine nuts, and a sprinkle of Parmesan, on the table in minutes with a little prep work. You'll cherish how the fresh, dynamic broccoli gets punched up with fiery stew chips and a solid hit of lemon juice, in addition to the stunning, rich kind of toasted pine nuts.

Ingredients:

- 2 tablespoons olive oil
- 1-pound broccoli florets
- 2 tablespoons unsalted spread
- 1 teaspoon minced garlic
- Salt and freshly ground black pepper
- 1/2 teaspoon ground lemon zing
- 2 tablespoons pine nuts, toasted
- 1 to 2 tablespoons fresh lemon juice

Method:

- Preheat oven to 500°F.

- In a big bowl, throw the broccoli with the oil and salt, and pepper to taste.
- Mastermind the florets in a solitary layer on a preparing sheet and meal, turning once, for 12 minutes, or until simply delicate.
- In the meantime, in a little pot, soften the spread over medium heat.
- Add the garlic and lemon zing and heat, blending, for around 1 moment.
- Let cool somewhat and mix in the lemon juice.
- Spot the broccoli in a serving bowl, pour the lemon margarine over it and throw to cover.
- Dissipate the toasted pine nuts over the top and serve.

15: The Easiest Hard-Boiled Eggs

Hard-bubbled eggs are an extraordinary food to have available as their uses are so adaptable. In addition to the fact that they are too delectable all alone, yet they're incredible in sandwiches, cleaved up on a salad, and the establishment for all devilled eggs. The secret to incredible hard-bubbled eggs isn't over-cooking them, which can leave a dim ring around the yolk and make their surface somewhat rubbery.

Ingredients:

- 1 tbsp. Sea salt
- 4 cups Water (or enough to cover eggs in the oven)
- 8 big Egg (or any number you need)
- 1 tbsp. Apple juice vinegar (or white if not paleo)

Method:

- Spot your crude eggs in a medium pan and cover with at least 2 creeps of cold water.
- Add 1 tablespoon of salt.
- Spot the dish over high heat until it arrives at a bubble.
- Mood killer heat, cover, and let it sit for 13 minutes.
- After precisely 13 minutes, eliminate the eggs from the dish and spot them in an ice-water shower and let them cool for five minutes.
- Cautiously break the eggs shells (ensuring most of the shell is broken).
- Delicately start eliminating the shells. The ice-water shower will "stun" the film in the middle of the egg-white and the eggshell, releasing the shell and permitting you to strip it off in almost one piece.
- Depending on the situation, you can plunge the egg (as you are stripping it) all through the water to eliminate any bits of the shell.
- Serve promptly, use in a recipe, or store in your fridge for three days.

16: Turkish Egg Breakfast

Turkish eggs recipe creates the ideal breakfast. Turkish Menemen Recipe is an incredibly delectable breakfast recipe. Summer tomatoes and green peppers consolidate with eggs in a container to simplify this, fast, and very yummy supper.

Ingredients:

- 2 tsp lemon juice
- 1 garlic clove, squashed

- 200g/7oz Greek-style plain yogurt
- 1 tsp ocean salt pieces
- 2 tbsp. unsalted spread
- 1 tsp Aleppo pepper
- 1 tbsp. extra virgin olive oil
- 2 huge free-roaming eggs, ice chest cold
- thick sourdough toast, to serve
- barely any fronds fresh dill, cleaved

Method:

- Top a pan off to 4cm/1½in profound with water and bring to the bubble.
- Spot the yogurt into a heatproof bowl sufficiently big to sit over the oven and mix in the garlic and salt.
- Spot the bowl over the oven, ensuring the base doesn't contact the water.
- Mix until it arrives at the internal heat level and has the consistency of softly whipped twofold cream.
- Mood killer the heat, leaving the bowl over the dish.
- Dissolve the spread tenderly in a different little pan until it is simply starting to turn hazelnut-earthy colored.
- Turn the heat off, then mix in the oil, trailed by the Aleppo pepper, and put in a safe spot.
- Fill a wide, lidded pot with 4cm/1½in water and spot over medium heat. Line a big plate with kitchen paper.
- Break the initial egg into a little fine-network sifter suspended over a little bowl, then lift and twirl

delicately for around 30 seconds, giving the watery piece of the white trickle access to the bowl; dispose of.

- Delicately tip the egg into a little cup or ramekin and pour 1 teaspoon of lemon juice onto it, focusing on the white. Rehash with the subsequent egg.
- At the point when the poaching water is simply beginning to stew, tenderly slide in the eggs, one on each side of the oven.
- Turn the heat directly down so there is no development in the water, and poach the eggs for 3–4 minutes, until the whites are set and the yolks still runny.
- Move the eggs to the lined plate utilizing an opened spoon.
- Separation the warm, rich yogurt between two shallow dishes, top each with a poached egg, pour over the peppery spread, dissipate the slashed dill on top and eat with the toast.

17: Veggie lover Coconut Kefir Banana Muffins

Simple to make, with simple ingredients, these clammy vegetarian banana biscuits are a pleasant base for fruit, nuts, and even chocolate chips. Blend and match your number one extra items to make your form utilizing our recipe as a format. Eat these biscuits warm with vegetarian margarine and natural product for breakfast, with nut spread for a protein-stuffed bite, or with a scoop of veggie lover frozen yogurt for a simple and tasty pastry.

Ingredients:

- 1 cup oats
- 1 tsp. vanilla concentrate
- 3 bananas
- 3 tbsp. maple syrup
- 1 cup coconut milk
- 1 tsp. heating pop
- 2 tsp. heating powder
- ½ cup slashed walnuts
- 2 tbsp. chipped or destroyed coconut
- 1 ¼ cups whole wheat flour + ¼ cup coconut flour

Method:

- Preheat oven to 350.
- Line 12 biscuit tins with papers. In a medium blending bowl, blend oats, flour(s), heating pop, and preparing powder.
- In a different bowl, pound bananas well with a fork or potato masher.
- Add vanilla, maple syrup, and coconut milk.
- Whisk everything together well, and afterward adds to dry ingredients. Blend until just mixed.
- Overlay in walnuts.
- A split blend between biscuit tins.
- Sprinkle biscuit tops with coconut.
- Prepare 23-27 minutes, or until tops simply start to firm and coconut starts to brown.

18: Turmeric Tofu Scramble

Tofu can be scary, yet this flexible plant protein takes on whatever flavor you give it. With each chomp of this exquisite scramble recipe, you'll feel better and stimulated. This morning meal will likewise help deal with your glucose levels. This turmeric tofu scramble is made with delightful, supplement-pressed flavors and is an amazing plant-based option in contrast to your commonplace egg-driven lunch.

Ingredients:

- 1 teaspoon turmeric powder
- 2 tablespoons healthful yeast (optional)
- 1/4 teaspoon cayenne pepper
- freshly ground black pepper (MUST)
- 2 tablespoons non-dairy milk or Veganaise
- grapeseed oil for cooking
- 1/2 teaspoon fine ocean salt
- 1/2 bundle (15 oz.) natural firm tofu (grew is extraordinary as well)

Method:

- Channel the tofu from the water and break the tofu into little scraps.
- Add the nourishing yeast, turmeric, pepper, salt, and milk, and mix well.
- Heat nonstick skillet on a low heat, then add oil.

- Add the tofu into the skillet and cook for around 3-4 minutes mixing sporadically.
- Add the child spinach and cover with a top to permit the heat to steam the spinach.
- Turn the heat off when you do this and reveal and two or multiple times more.
- Serve hot with cherry tomatoes and avocado toast. (red peppers or different veggies likewise work incredibly, however, tomatoes are a lot speedier to cook and the concentration here is 5 minutes.

19: Shredded Brussels Sprouts with Bacon and Onions

Shredded Brussels sprouts are my #1 fresh dish, truly give me a fork. It's a side dish that meets up super-quick. Each chomp is stacked with flavor, toss with garlic, and finished off with a firm, smoky bacon. It makes the whole cycle a lot simpler and truly shreds the fledglings into a flawless knot of green. You can likewise utilize a sharp blade and get the cuts as slim as could be expected.

Ingredients:

- 4 cups chicken stock or low-sodium stock
- Coarse salt and freshly ground pepper
- 1 Spanish onion, daintily cut
- 8 garlic cloves, split the long way
- 4 pounds Brussels sprouts, managed
- 1/2 pound thickly cut lean bacon, cut across into flimsy strips
- Sugar (optional)

Method:

- In a big, profound skillet, cook the bacon over tolerably high heat until caramelized, around 8 minutes.
- Add the onion and garlic, reduce the heat to direct, and cook, mixing, until relaxed, around 5 minutes.
- Add the stock, season with salt and pepper and a spot of sugar, and cook until the fluid has reduced to 1 cup, around 12 minutes.
- Then, in a large pot of bubbling salted water, whiten the Brussels sprouts until scarcely delicate, around 3 minutes.
- Add the fledglings to the skillet. Stew delicately over moderate heat, mixing every so often, until delicate all through, around 10 minutes; season with salt and pepper.
- Utilizing an opened spoon, move to a bowl.
- Heat the fluid in the skillet over tolerably high heat until reduced to 1/2 cup. Pour the sauce over the Brussels fledglings and serve.

20: Vegan Coconut Kefir Banana Muffins

These biscuits taste natural and consoling, given their feathery, banana-mixed internal parts. They're also fun and tropical, because of the Shredded coconut you'll discover within and on the biscuit tops. A little lemon zing unites every one of the flavors.

These biscuits are improved with essentially ready bananas, with simply a trace of coconut palm sugar (or brown sugar).

If you don't have these elective flours available, simply supplant them with wheat or gluten-free flour of your decision. With just 10 ingredients, these sound, plant-based biscuits are not difficult to heat up, and they will be a certain fire hit with the whole family.

Ingredients:

- ½ cup virgin coconut oil, dissolved
- ¼ cup honey
- 1 ½ teaspoon preparing powder
- ¼ teaspoon fine ocean salt
- ½ cup white whole wheat flour or ordinary whole wheat flour
- ¾ cup unsweetened Shredded coconut, isolated
- 1 tablespoon turbinado (crude) sugar
- ½ teaspoon lemon zing (the zing from about ½ medium lemon)
- 1 cup squashed ready banana (from around 3 bananas)
- 1 big egg, ideally at room temperature
- 1 teaspoon vanilla concentrate
- ¾ cup whole wheat baked good flour or white/standard whole wheat flour

Method:

- Preheat stove to 375 degrees Fahrenheit. If important, oil every one of the 12 cups of your biscuit tin with spread or biscuit liners (my dish is non-stick and didn't need any oil).

- In a medium bowl, whisk together the flours, salt, heating powder, and lemon zing. Mix in ½ cup of the shredded coconut.
- In a different, medium bowl, whisk together the pounded banana, honey, coconut oil, egg, and vanilla.
- Empty the wet ingredients into the dry ingredients and mix until just consolidated.
- Separation the player uniformly between the biscuit cups (a meager ¼ cup hitter every), then sprinkle the biscuit tops with the excess ¼ cup Shredded coconut.
- Sprinkle the tops with crude sugar.
- Prepare for around 17 to 20 minutes, until a toothpick embedded into the middle, tells the truth.
- Move biscuits to a cooling rack and let them cool.

21: Avocado Ricotta Power Toast

This avocado toast gets a novel turn with extra garnishes of lemon ricotta, kale microgreens, and a sprinkle of all that bagel zest. This ricotta avocado toast is uncommonly acceptable, getting its splendid, fresh taste from the lemony ricotta. The pillowy ricotta shapes the base for the avocado which gets finished off with a runny egg for additional flavor. Polished off with a sprinkling of fragile microgreens and a sprinkle of all that bagel zest, this toast shines a different light on the words simple, workday breakfast.

Ingredients:

- 4 eggs
- 6 tablespoons ricotta cheddar

- 3 avocados, crushed
- 4 tablespoons harissa
- 4 cups of whole wheat, toasted
- 1/4 cup cut green onions
- 1 teaspoon white vinegar

Method:

- Fill a big skillet around 1/2″ loaded with water.
- Heat to the point of boiling.
- Add bread to toaster oven and toast until somewhat sautéed.
- Eliminate and let sit.
- Add a sprinkle of white vinegar to the bubbling water (around 1 teaspoon).
- Quickly include 4 eggs separating them. Cover.
- Turn burners off.
- Leave eggs covered with the heat off for 4-5 minutes.
- Meanwhile, add 1/2 tablespoons of ricotta to each piece of toast, just as 1/4 cup of squashed avocado, and 1 tablespoon of harissa.
- When eggs poached.
- Delicately eliminate from water (make certain to empty any fluid of the skillet) and spot on top of amassed toast.
- Embellishment with green onions.
- Serve!

Burgers will consistently be one of my #1 food varieties! These Completely Vegan Lentil Burgers permit you to appreciate this exemplary fave yet in a MUCH better manner! Every burger contains such a lot of plant-based goodness; your body will much be obliged.

These fiery Vegan Lentil Burgers are made with split red lentils and are finished off with the most delectable rich vegetarian avocado sauce. Prepared in less than 20 minutes, these lentil patties are extraordinary as burgers, lettuce wraps, or in a salad.

Ingredients:

- 1 onion, slashed
- ½ pound (227 g) of mushrooms, freshly cut
- 2 tablespoons (30 mL) of vegetable oil
- 2 cups (500 mL) of cooked lentils
- 4 cloves of garlic, freshly slashed
- 1 cup (250 mL) of bread morsels
- 2 tablespoons (30 mL) of dried thyme
- ½ cup (125 mL) of nut or almond margarine
- ¼ cup (60 mL) of chia seeds
- 2 tablespoons (30 mL) of miso glue
- 2 tablespoons (30 mL) of soy sauce
- 2 cups (500 mL) of yam, ground

Method:

- Sprinkle the oil into your skillet over medium-high heat.
- Toss in the mushrooms, onion, and garlic, and sauté until they become brown and tasty around 10 minutes. Move the mix to your food processor.
- Add every one of the excess ingredients except the ground yam. Puree the combination until everything is easily joined.
- Move the combination to a mixing bowl and mix in the yam by hand so it doesn't separate in the machine.
- Rest the combination for ten minutes, giving the chia seeds time to do something amazing.
- Utilizing your hands, shape the mix into equally framed patties.
- They might be cooked promptly, refrigerated for a few days, or frozen for a month.
- When the time has come to cook you have heaps of alternatives for these burgers.
- You may broil them in a daintily oiled sauté skillet on your burner, singe them on your iron, barbecue, or BBQ, or even prepare in your broiler at 400°F (200°C) for 15 to 20 minutes.
- Whatever method you pick, remember that these burgers brown moderately rapidly so medium-high heat will permit the focuses to keep up while the outsides cook.

23: Baked Mahi Mahi

It's an incredible, more affordable option in contrast to halibut, and can be barbecued, cooked, or even singed. Yet, one of our number one different ways to set it up is to just dish burn it, which lets the flavors and flaky surface sparkle. Singing it in a skillet also allows you to make a rich, lemony sauce to shower everywhere on the fish. All you need to finish this simple fish meal is a green salad or vegetable, and possibly some bread or rice to sop up all that delectable sauce. Here's the simplest method to cook mahi mahi.

Ingredients:

- ¼ tsp salt
- ¾ cup cream
- ¼ tsp pepper
- ½ cup raspberry juice
- ¼ cup balsamic vinegar
- 1 tbsp. spread
- 6-piece medium size mahi-mahi

Method:

- Spread 1 tablespoon of margarine on 6 bits of medium-sized mahi-mahi and sprinkle it with 1/4 teaspoon every one of pepper and salt.
- Orchestrate the fishes on a lubed heating dish. Pour 3/4 cup of cream and 1/4 cup of Balsamic vinegar over the fish.

- Cover the heating dish with material paper and spot it inside a broiler that has been preheated to 450 degrees Fahrenheit. Cook for 12 minutes.

24: Grass-Fed Burgers

If you've changed to grass-took care of meat, you likely realize that it's liberated from chemicals and lower in fat, and higher in some significant supplements than ordinary grain-took care of hamburger. If you bought it simply from a limited-scale farmer, you may likewise be aware of subtleties like the cows' variety and age.

Ingredients:

- 4 teaspoons fit salt
- 2 lbs. Belcampo ground hamburger
- 4 Slices provolone cheddar
- 8 Slices cooked bacon
- 4 Brioche burger buns
- 4 Slices tomato and other burger garnishes (pickles, red onion)

Method:

- Separation 2 lbs. grass-took care of hamburger into four segments.
- To not exhaust the meat, eliminate it from the bundle and simply shape it into burger patties around 5" across – don't massage the meat.
- Sprinkle every burger with one teaspoon Kosher salt partitioned one half on each side

- Preheat barbecue on high
- Cook for 3 minutes on each side for Medium Rare, 4 minutes on each side for Medium. Eliminate from heat when inner temp arrives at 125F.
- Spot cheddar on the burger after the main flip
- Eliminate from the flame broil and spot on a bun with garnish and cooked Bacon

25: Cinnamon Roll Fat Bombs

The cinnamon fat bombs are made keto-accommodating by keeping the ingredients low carb and high fat, and the cream cheddar icing is amazingly acceptable. This is genuinely a high-fat keto bite that is amazing. Here's a recipe for making cinnamon simply move fat bombs.

Ingredients:

- ½ cup almond flour
- ½ cup unsalted margarine, at room temperature
- 1 tsp ground cinnamon
- 3 ½ tbsp. granulated Stevia or another granulated sugar to taste
- For cream cheddar icing:
- ½ tsp vanilla concentrate
- 3 tbsp. cream cheddar
- 1 ½ tbsp. substantial cream
- 1 ½ tbsp. granulated Stevia or another granulated low carb sugar to taste

Method:

- In a bowl place the spread and granulated Stevia and utilizing an electric mixer beat on medium speed until mixed.
- Add the almond flour and cinnamon and beat to consolidate.
- Cover the batter and refrigerate for 30 minutes or until adequately hard to frame balls.
- Free the mixture once again from the fridge and fold into balls around 1 tablespoon in size.
- Freeze the balls for 20 minutes.
- To make the icing, in a microwave-safe bowl join every one of the ingredients.
- Microwave on high for 20 seconds.
- Eliminate from the microwave and mix.
- Shower the icing over the balls.
- Keep the balls in a water/airproof holder in the fridge until prepared to serve.

26: Cauliflower Popcorn

This low-carb cauliflower popcorn is perhaps the yummiest (and generally fun!) approach to eat cauliflower. No spongy business here! With its wonderfully firm covering, this dish is a hit with the whole family, if they are watching their carbs. Functions admirably as finger food, as an hors d'oeuvre, or as a side dish.

Ingredients:

- 1 cup (75g) panko breadcrumbs
- 1 teaspoon smoked paprika
- 1 Coles Australian Free Range Egg, delicately whisked
- 2 teaspoons coarsely chopped thyme twigs
- 1 cauliflower, cut into little florets
- 1/2 cup (40g) finely ground parmesan

Method:

- Preheat stove to 200°C. Line a preparing plate with heating paper.
- Cook the cauliflower in a big pot of bubbling water for 5 mins or until simply delicate. Channel well.
- Move to a big bowl. Mix in the egg.
- Consolidate the breadcrumbs, parmesan, paprika, and thyme in a big bowl. Add the cauliflower mix and toss to join.
- Mastermind the mix in a solitary layer over the lined plate. Shower well with olive oil splash. Season.

27: Best Baked Potato

This heated potato recipe is pretty much as a clear record as it gets. Don't hesitate to add different flavors to the salt-and-pepper mix, like cumin or smoked paprika, and get done with whatever cheddar you like. In case you're utilizing little potatoes, you can slice them down the middle or if they're minuscule, you can simply give them a little jab with a fork or blade before preparing to permit the steam to getaway.

Ingredients:

- 1/4 cup olive oil
- 1 tablespoon salt
- 4 big Russet potatoes

Method:

- Preheat the stove to 425 degrees.
- Wash and dry the potatoes.
- Puncture the potato 2-3 times with a fork
- Rub oil everywhere on the potatoes (or pick one of the different alternatives above to rub outwardly).
- Rub salt everywhere on the potatoes. We incline toward coarse ocean salt or pink Himalayan salt.
- Spot the potatoes on a preparing sheet and heat for around 45 minutes.
- The specific preparing time will rely upon how big the potatoes are. The potato ought to be delicate inside if you stick a fork into it.
- Present with spread, chives, cheddar, sharp cream, and the entirety of your #1 garnishes!

28: Crispy Cauliflower Pizza Crust

Cauliflower Pizza Crust is extremely popular however if you don't make it effectively, it tends to be a spongy disillusionment. The objective is to have a decent firm hull, not a limp, soft wreck. After much experimentation, we at last sorted out the key to the whole fresh Cauliflower Pizza Crust.

This cauliflower pizza outside layer recipe utilizes basic ingredients with the goal that you can the entirety of the tasty garnishes you like. It's low carb, gluten-free, without grain, and pressing the flavor. This is what you'll have to make it:

Ingredients:

- 2 pounds' cauliflower florets riced
- 1 egg beaten
- 1 teaspoon dried oregano
- 1/4 teaspoon Himalayan salt
- 1/2 cup ground mozzarella cheddar or Parmesan cheddar

Method:

- Preheat stove to 400 degrees F.
- Heartbeat bunches of crude cauliflower florets in a food processor, until a rice-like surface, is accomplished. However, don't over-cycle or cream it.
- Microwave the cauliflower rice for around 1 moment or until delicate. Or heat it: In a large pot, load up with about an inch of water, and heat it to the point of boiling.
- Add the cauliflower "rice" and cover. Cook around 4-5 minutes. After the cauliflower is cooked, channel it into a fine sifter or over cheesecloth.
- On your counter over a towel, spread out a fine-network cheesecloth.
- Pour the mix on the cheesecloth and utilizing the cheesecloth, assemble and press out any additional dampness into the sink.

- Pat much more dampness out by tapping again with the towel. Ensure all the water is taken out by crushing out on the towel.
- Whenever dampness is taken out, move "rice" to a large mixing bowl. Add beaten egg, cheddar, oregano, and salt. You may have to utilize your hands to mix.
- Press the mixture out onto a heating sheet fixed with material paper.
- Utilizing hands press level and crush in the sides to frame a shape at ⅓ inch high. Make marginally higher on the sides.
- Heat 35-40 minutes at 400 degrees F or until the outside layer is firm and amazing brown.
- Eliminate from broiler and add garnishes.
- Heat an extra 5-10 minutes until cheddar is hot and effervescent. Serve right away.

29: Almond Apple Spice Muffins

These paleo apple biscuits are so fast and simple to assemble thus great! Heat them toward the end of the week and freeze for in and out morning meals during the week. They're gluten-free and without grain with a sans dairy alternative.

Ingredients:

- 1 teaspoon allspice
- 1 teaspoon cloves
- 2 cups almond meal
- 4 eggs
- 1 cup unsweetened fruit purée

- 5 scoops of vanilla protein powder
- 1/2 stick margarine
- 1 tablespoon cinnamon

Method:

- Preheat the broiler to 350 degrees. Liquefy margarine in the microwave (~30 seconds on low heat).
- Completely mix every one of the ingredients in a bowl.
- Splash biscuit tin with non-stick cooking shower or use cupcake liners.
- Empty mix into biscuit tins, make a point, not to overload (~3/4 full); this should make 12 biscuits (2 biscuit plate).
- Spot one plate in the broiler and cook for 12 minutes.
- Make a point not to overcook as the biscuits will turn out to be extremely dry.
- When cooked, eliminate from the broiler and cook the second biscuit plate.

30: Healthy Mexican Fried Rice

This Mexican singed rice recipe is also an extraordinary method to rapidly make a side dish utilizing precooked rice from a clump cooking meeting or extra rice. The way to making incredible singed rice is utilizing cooked, cold rice. When I make any kind of singed rice recipe, I like to clump cook rice the other day and refrigerate it short-term so it gets quite cold. Cooked rice also freezes well if you needed to make a bigger group and freeze it in the sums you need for this and other rice plans.

Ingredients:

- 2 teaspoons olive oil
- 100 grams (1/2 cup) brown rice
- 1 little yellow onion, sliced
- 1 garlic clove, squashed
- 1 little bean stew pepper, deseeded and chopped
- 1 teaspoon Mexican stew powder
- 1/2 can corn portions
- 1/2 can black beans, washed
- 1 tablespoon fresh lime juice
- 100-gram grape tomatoes, chopped
- Fresh coriander, to serve
- Lime wedges, to serve
- 60-gram feta disintegrated
- 1/4 little red onion, finely slashed
- 1/2 little avocado, quartered and cut

Method:

- Cook the rice in a large pan of bubbling water for 25 minutes or until delicate.
- Channel well, then spread onto a large plate and spot into the ice chest, uncovered, for at any rate 60 minutes.
- Heat the oil in a big griddle over medium heat.
- Add the yellow onion and stew pepper, and cook for five minutes or until delicate. Add the garlic and bean stew powder.

- Proceed to cook and mix for 30 seconds or until fragrant.
- Add the rice and cook, mixing, for two minutes until softly seared and all around joined with the onion mix.
- Add the beans and corn and keep cooking, mixing regularly, until warmed through. Pour lime squeeze over and toss to consolidate.
- Consolidate the tomatoes and red onion and season to taste.
- Split the rice mix between serving bowls and top with the tomato combination, feta, avocado, coriander, and lime wedges.

31: Turkey Tacos

Here is another best recipe for your lunch. This recipe has a couple of stunts at its disposal to ensure each chomp is delicious and completely prepared. Coming to tortillas close to you in around 15 minutes.

Ingredients:

- 8 taco shells
- 1 tablespoon olive oil
- 1-pound ground turkey
- 1 little yellow onion, slashed
- ½ teaspoon bean stew powder
- Salt
- 1 ½ cups (6 ounces) shredded Cheddar
- 1 little head of romaine lettuce, Shredded
- 1 beefsteak tomato, cubed

Method:

- Heat the oil in a medium heat.
- Add the onion and cook, mixing, until marginally delicate, around 4 minutes.
- Add the turkey and cook, disintegrating with the rear of a spoon, until no hint of pink remaining parts, 5 to 7 minutes.
- Mix in the bean stew powder and ½ teaspoon salt.
- Spoon the filling into the taco shells and top with lettuce, Cheddar, and tomato.

32: Healthy Spaghetti Bolognese

Making hand-crafted bolognese sauce is simpler than you'd suspect! This healthy bolognese is a delectable, flavorful dish that you can make without any preparation in just 25 minutes.

Ingredients:

- 2 garlic cloves, stripped and finely sliced
- 1 tsp light olive oil
- 1 medium onion, finely sliced
- 1 medium courgette, finely cubed
- 1 celery sticks, finely sliced
- 600ml meat stock
- 400g turkey mince
- 1 big carrot, ground
- 2 sound leaves
- 300g whole-wheat spaghetti
- 150ml red wine (optional)

- 400g tin sliced tomatoes
- Parmesan shavings, to serve
- basil leaves, to serve

Method:

- Heat the oil in a big, non-stick, weighty lined pan.
- Add the onion, celery, and 2 tablespoons water and fry for 5 minutes or until the vegetables have mellowed.
- Add the courgette and fry for another 2-3 minutes.
- Add the mince and garlic and fry for another 3-4 minutes, mixing now and again or until the mince has separated and is beginning to brown. Mix well.
- Add the ground carrot and 150ml of the hamburger stock or red wine, whenever liked, and stew for 3-4 minutes.
- Then add the tinned tomatoes, 450ml hamburger stock, and the narrows leaves and bring them to the heat.
- Cover with a top, turn down the heat to medium-low, and leave to stew for 45 minutes, mixing once in a while.
- Eliminate the cover and cook for another 10-15 minutes, or until the fluid has reduced and thickened to wanted consistency.
- Cook the spaghetti as per parcel directions, channel, and split between 6 plates. Spot a spoonful of Bolognese on top of each plate, dissipate with basil leaves and Parmesan shavings.

The trail mix nibble recipe I am showing you today is exceptionally healthy since it is wealthy in cancer prevention agents. As you may know, cell reinforcements advance great wellbeing as they help stay away from infections. All the more explicitly, cancer prevention agents help hinder the oxidation of cells in our body.

When cells oxidize, they create free extremists, which are otherwise called cell bi-items. It is protected to have a sensible measure of these free revolutionaries in the body. Notwithstanding, when the free revolutionaries are in abundance, they can unleash ruin on our organic entity's cell mechanical assembly.

Ingredients:

- Cheerios
- Wheat, corn, or rice Chex cereal
- Low-fat popcorn
- Low-fat granola cereal bunches
- Low-fat sesame seeds
- Unsalted pretzel winds or sticks
- Unsalted sunflower seeds (shelled)
- Sans sugar chocolate chips or M&Ms
- Soy nuts
- Unsalted scaled-down rice cakes

Method:

- You can likewise buy low sugar or sans sugar dried fruit at different wellbeing food stores.
- Likewise, one of the most reduced sugar-dried fruits is apple.
- Figs are another healthy decision.
- If you should utilize high glossed-over treats, use them with some restraint.
- While setting up these treats, you can toss them in close Ziploc baggies that are not difficult to bring on picnics, strolls, or any place you go.

34: Weight Watchers Berry Crisp

This Weight Watchers Berry Crisp is a delightful and simple sweet you don't need to feel remorseful about enjoying. This fast, 5-ingredient treat hits every one of the spots of those old top choices yet with way fewer calories. The recipe is made with fresh berries and improved with a dash of brown sugar and a trace of cinnamon. It's done off with a fresh ingredient made of low-fat granola.

Ingredients:

- 1½ cups raspberries
- 1½ cups fresh blackberries
- 1½ cups blueberries
- ¾ cup generally useful flour

- ¼ cup sugar
- ½ cup amazing brown sugar, stuffed
- ¾ cup moved oats
- ½ teaspoon cinnamon
- Fat-free frozen vanilla yogurt, optional
- ½ cup reduced-fat margarine, cold
- Gently whipped cream, optional

Method:

- Preheat broiler to 350 degrees
- In a medium bowl utilizing an elastic spatula, delicately toss together the blackberries, raspberries, blueberries, and white sugar; put in a safe spot
- In a different medium bowl, join flour, oats, brown sugar, and cinnamon. Add the margarine in pieces and cautiously mix while keeping brittle.
- Coat 6 (3 ½-inch) ramekins with a cooking splash, see prep tip. Split the sugared berries between them.
- Separation and sprinkle equitably absurd the disintegrate mix, about ⅓ cup for each.
- Line a preparing sheet with material paper or foil. Spot the 6 ramekin cups on the skillet.
- Prepare for around 40 minutes until amazing brown. Top with a little whipped cream or frozen yogurt, whenever wanted.

35: San Choy Bau Bowl

San Choy Bau is one of those dishes my children continue to request over and over. It's an incredible one for outdoors in the light of the fact that the ingredients store effectively (clam sauce ought to be kept in the refrigerator), and you just need one skillet. A similar sum functions as a starter for a large gathering (diamond lettuce goes home better for this) – or feed the family as a simple without carb lunch.

Ingredients:

- 500g pork mince
- 1 tablespoon ground ginger
- 1/4 cup clam sauce
- 2 garlic cloves, finely slashed
- 1 tablespoon nut oil
- 2 tablespoons kecap manis
- 2 teaspoons lime juice
- 1/2 tablespoon caster sugar
- 1 teaspoon sesame oil
- coriander leaves
- 1 little chunk of ice lettuce
- salted carrots
- singed shallots
- 1/4 cup slashed peanuts, gently cooked with salt

Method:

- Heat the nut oil in a wok over high heat.

- Add the pork mince, garlic, and ginger to the wok and cook through. Channel off any fluid to guarantee the mince is very dry.
- In a little bowl join the shellfish sauce, caster sugar, kecap manis, lime juice, and sesame oil.
- Add 66% of the sauce to the pork mince and mix through a few minutes until the sauce thickens.
- Eliminate the wok from the heat and permit the mince to cool marginally.
- In a little, dry fry container, toast the peanuts and put them to the side to cool.
- Wash, dry, and trim your lettuce leaves and spread them out on a plate.
- Split the mince combination between the lettuce cups.
- Top each San Choy Bau with salted carrot, broiled peanuts, coriander leaves, and seared shallots.
- Spoon over the leftover sauce.

To make a sheet dish form of this exemplary meal, broil the potatoes until delicate and afterward cook everything under the oven to give it an amazing brown burn. Sheet Pan Steak and Potatoes conveys all the generous solace however practically no dishes to tidy up.

Ingredients:

- 1 head of broccoli, cut into florets
- 1/4 cup olive oil
- 2 tablespoons fresh rosemary, minced (or 2 teaspoons dry, squashed)
- 2 tablespoons balsamic vinegar
- Fit salt
- 9 cloves garlic, minced and isolated
- Fresh broke black pepper
- 1/2 pounds Yukon gold potatoes, split
- 2 pounds of level iron steak (can substitute flank steak simply try to check the inward temp)

Method:

- Preheat broiler to 450°. Line a large rimmed heating sheet with foil.
- Spot the steak in a large zipper-top pack with the 1/4 cup olive oil, 4 cloves of garlic, salt, vinegar, balsamic and pepper.

- Go to cover and let marinate at any rate 1 hour as long as 8 hours.
- Disperse potatoes and rosemary on the heating sheet and shower with 1 tablespoon of olive oil, and season with salt and pepper.
- Toss tenderly with utensils to cover and spread them out equitably.
- Cook potatoes mix until they start to brown around the edges, around 20 minutes.
- Join the leftover 2 tablespoons of olive oil, broccoli, and remaining garlic in a bowl; season with salt and pepper, and toss to cover. Spot on the heating sheet alongside the potatoes.
- Spot an ovenproof wire rack over the broccoli and potatoes. Eliminate the steak from the zip-top sack and shake off the abundance marinade. Lay the steak on the rack.
- Return the preparing sheet to the broiler and dish until a moment read thermometer embedded evenly into the focal point of meat registers 125, around 10 to 15 minutes.
- Eliminate from the broiler and let rest for 5 to 10 minutes before cutting.

37: Poached Eggs and Avocado Toasts

Make the most of your day away from work with a nutritious and healthy lunch with this Avocado Toast with Poached Egg. A basic simple avocado concoction spread on a cut of toasted wholegrain bread and finished off with a poached egg. It is flavorful. This fair may turn into a customary thing on your lunch menu.

You need a wonderfully ready avocado and a pleasant thick cut of fresh bread to toast. Since avocados become brown when the fruit is presented to the air, pound it up with a little lemon squeeze then sprinkle some salt in to draw out the flavor.

Ingredients:

- 2 eggs
- salt and pepper for ingredient
- 2 cups of wholegrain bread
- 2 tablespoons shaved Parmesan cheddar
- quartered treasure tomatoes for serving
- fresh spices (parsley, thyme, or basil) for ingredient
- 1/3 avocado (for the most part I cut it down the middle yet don't utilize every last bit of it. alright fine perhaps I do.)

Method:

- Carry a pot of water to heat (utilize sufficient water to cover the eggs when they lay in the base).

- Drop the metal edges (external edge just) of two artisan container covers into the pot so they are laying level on the base.
- When the water is bubbling, turn off the heat and cautiously break the eggs simply into each edge.
- Cover the pot and poach for 5 minutes (4 for too delicate, 4:30 for delicate, at least 5 for semi-delicate yolks).
- While the eggs are cooking, toast the bread and crush the avocado on each piece of toast.
- When the eggs are done, utilize a spatula to lift the eggs out of the water. Delicately remove the edge from the eggs (I do this privilege on the spatula, over the water) and spot the poached eggs on top of the toast.
- Sprinkle with Parmesan cheddar, salt, pepper, and fresh spices; present with the fresh quartered legacy tomatoes.

Chapter: 3 Salad & Soups

38: Veggie-Packed Cheesy Chicken Salad

These veggie-pressed dinners will have you covered from breakfast to dinner. Furthermore, these plans have close to 15 grams of sugars for every serving. Plans like Green Shakshuka and Buffalo Chicken Cauliflower Pizza are vivid, scrumptious, and brimming with supplements and nutrients.

Ingredients:

- 1 lb. uncooked slight cut chicken breasts
- 7 tablespoons diminished fat balsamic vinaigrette dressing
- 1 medium zucchini (8 oz.), cut the long way down the middle
- 1 medium red onion, cut into 1/4-inch cuts
- 4 plum (Roma) tomatoes, cut down the middle
- 6 cups torn arugula
- ½ cup disintegrated feta cheddar (2 oz.)

Method:

- Heat gas or charcoal barbecue. Brush chicken with 1 tablespoon of the dressing. Cautiously brush oil on the barbecue rack.
- Spot chicken, zucchini, and onion on flame broil over medium heat.

- Cover flame broil; cook 8 to 10 minutes, turning once, until chicken is not, at this point pink in focus and vegetables are delicate.
- Add tomato parts to flame broil throughout the previous 4 minutes of cooking.
- Reduce chicken and vegetables from flame broil to cutting board.
- Cut chicken across into slender cuts; coarsely cleave vegetables.
- In a large bowl, throw chicken, vegetables, and the leftover 6 tablespoons of dressing.
- Add arugula and cheddar; throw tenderly. Serve right away.

39: Cobb Salad with Brown Derby Dressing

The recipe contained in this Cobb Salad with French Dressing was given to me by Walt Disney World Guest Services or a Disney Chef at the eatery. The recipe in Cobb Salad with French Dressing may have been downsized by the Disney Chefs for the home culinary specialist. We love this salad. It's expensive even by Disney principles yet it genuinely is scrumptious.

Salad ingredients:

- 1/2 package watercress
- 3 eggs, hard-cooked
- 1/2 head icy mass lettuce
- 1 little pack chicory
- 2 medium tomatoes, whitened and stripped

- 1/2 head romaine lettuce
- 1/2 cups cooked turkey breast, cubed
- 2 tablespoons slashed chives
- 6 strips fresh bacon, disintegrated
- 1/2 cup blue cheddar, disintegrated

French Dressing Ingredients:

- 1/2 teaspoon sugar
- 1/2 cup water
- 1/4 tablespoons salt
- 1 clove garlic, chopped
- 1/2 cups salad oil
- 1/2 cup red wine vinegar
- 1/2 teaspoons Worcestershire sauce
- Juice of 1/2 lemon
- 1/2 teaspoon English mustard
- 1/2 cup olive oil
- 1/2 tablespoon ground dark pepper

Method for Cobb Salad:

- Slash all greens fine and mastermind in a salad bowl.
- Cut tomatoes down the middle, reduce seeds, and dice fine.
- Likewise dice the turkey, avocado, and eggs.
- Mastermind the above ingredients, just as the blue cheddar and bacon disintegrate, in straight lines across the greens.

- Mastermind the chives slantingly across the above lines.
- Present the salad at the table, then throw it with the dressing.
- Spot on chilled plates with a watercress enhancement.

Method for Dressing:

- Mix all ingredients aside from oils.
- Then add olive oil and salad oils and blend well.
- Mix well again before blending in with the salad.

40: Speedy Thai Noodle Salad

Thai Noodle Salad with the BEST EVER Peanut Sauce-stacked up with sound veggies! This veggie lover salad is incredible for potlucks and Sunday dinner - prep and keeps going as long as 5 days in the refrigerator. Gluten-free versatile. Incorporates a 35-second video.

Ingredients:

- 4 cups blend of cabbage, carrots, and radish, destroyed or ground
- 6-ounce dry noodles (earthy colored rice noodles, cushion Thai style rice noodles, soba noodles, linguini)
- 3 scallions, cut
- 1 red chime pepper, finely cut
- ½ pack cilantro, chopped (or sub basil and mint)
- ¼–½ cup broiled, squashed peanuts (embellish)
- 1 tablespoon jalapeño (finely chopped)

Method:

- Cook pasta as per bearings on the package.
- Channel and chill under cool running water.
- Throw: Place destroyed veggies, chime pepper, scallions, cilantro, and jalapeño into a serving bowl. Throw.
- Add the chilly noodles to the serving bowl and throw once more. Pour the nut sauce up and over and throw well to join.
- (However you would prefer), add stew drops if you need and serve, decorating with broiled peanuts and cilantro and a lime wedge.

41: Warm Roasted Vegetable Farro Salad

If you're in the disposition for a dinner salad that is generous, solid, and heavenly, then look no farther than this Roasted Vegetable and Farro Salad. This salad joins nutty, chewy faro with an assortment of broiled vegetables, all threw in a balsamic vinaigrette and present with disintegrated feta.

Ingredients:

- ⅔ cup broccoli florets
- 1½ cups cooked farro
- ¼ cup grape tomatoes divided
- ½ of ringer pepper, chopped
- ¼ of zucchini, cubed
- 1 tsp olive oil
- 1 tsp ocean salt + more to taste
- 1 clove garlic, shredded
- 1 tsp dried or fresh rosemary

- 4-5 kalamata olives, cut
- 2 tbsp. disintegrated goat cheddar
- ¼ cup pecan parts, slashed

Method:

- Preheat the broiler to 400°F and fix a skillet with material paper.
- Throw broccoli, tomatoes, zucchini, and ringer pepper with olive oil, rosemary, salt, and shredded garlic in a bowl until equally covered.
- Spread on arranged dish and meal in preheated broiler for 25 minutes.
- Joined broiled vegetables with cooked farro, cut olives, and pecans.
- Add salt to taste.
- Top with disintegrated goat cheddar and serve.

42: Cajun Potato, Shrimp, and Avocado Salad

We have another best recipe in our book that is Cajun Potato, Shrimp, and Avocado Salad. It is the best discontinuous fasting recipe to attempt. Many people like it and it is not difficult to make.

Ingredients:

- 2 spring onions (finely cut)
- 2 teaspoons Cajun preparing
- 1 garlic clove (shredded)
- 1 tablespoon oil (olive oil)
- 1 avocado (stripped, stoned, and cubed)

- 1 cup horse feed sprout
- Salt (to bubble potatoes)
- 300-gram potatoes (fresh potatoes, little child or talks 10 oz. divided)
- 250-gram crude shrimp (ruler prawns, 8 oz., cooked and stripped)

Method:

- Cook the potatoes in an enormous pot of delicately salted bubbling water for 10 to 15 minutes or until delicate, channel well.
- Heat the oil in a wok or large nonstick griddle/skillet.
- Add the prawns, garlic, spring onions, and Cajun preparing and pan sear for 2 to 3 minutes or until the prawns are hot.
- Mix in the potatoes and cook briefly.
- Move to serve dishes and top with the avocado and the hay fledglings and serve.

43: Simple Black Bean Soup

It is a basic and solid soup made with canned dark beans and regular ingredients! This delightful dark bean soup is veggie-lover, without gluten, and vegan. This soup is ideal for lunch, occupied weeknights, or taking care of an eager group. Our whole family cherishes this soup and we as a whole get energized when it's on the menu! It hits the recognize without fail.

Ingredients:

- 1 medium red onion, finely chopped
- 2 tbsp. extra-virgin olive oil
- 2 cloves garlic, shredded
- 1 tbsp. tomato glue
- 1 tbsp. shredded jalapeños
- salt
- 1 tsp. bean stew powder
- Freshly ground dark pepper
- 1/2 tsp. cumin
- 3 (15-oz.) jars dark beans, with fluid
- 1 bay leaf
- 1 qt. low-sodium chicken or vegetable stock
- acrid cream, for embellish
- Cleaved fresh cilantro, for embellish
- Cut avocado, to decorate

Method:

- In an enormous pot over medium heat, heat oil. Add onion and cook until delicate and clear, around 5 minutes.
- Add jalapeños and garlic and cook until fragrant, around 2 minutes.
- Add tomato glue, mix to cover vegetables, and cook about a brief more. Season with salt, bean stew powder, pepper, and cumin and mix to cover.
- Add dark beans with their fluid and chicken stock. Mix soup, add cove leaf and heat to the point of boiling.

- Quickly decrease to a stew and let stew until marginally diminished around 15 minutes. Reduce inlet leaf.
- Utilizing a drenching blender or food processor, mix the soup to wanted consistency.
- Present with a touch of sharp cream, cut avocado, and cilantro.

44: Chicken with Fried Cauliflower Rice

This Chicken Fried Cauliflower Rice is not difficult to make and can be filled in as your principal dish or as a side dish. It's low in focuses, low in carbs, and loaded up with veggies and protein. It is a fast and simple Asian one container supper recipe that the whole family will cherish.

Ingredients:

- 2 big eggs
- 1 tablespoon sesame oil
- 1/2 cup chopped onion
- 2 tablespoons olive or avocado oil
- 1 clove garlic, crushed
- 1 teaspoon fresh ginger, crushed
- 4 teaspoons soy sauce, separated
- 1 cup cooked chicken
- 1 pound riced cauliflower
- 1/2 cup chopped scallions
- 1 tablespoon stew glue

Method:

- Heat oil in a big oven or wok over medium heat.
- Add the onion and cook, mixing regularly, until clear.
- Add the ginger, garlic, and chicken to the container and keep cooking for 2 minutes.

- Add the cauliflower to the oven and sprinkle with 3 teaspoons (1 tablespoon) of soy sauce and stew glue.
- Mix well and cook for 3 minutes or until the cauliflower has mollified.
- Push the cauliflower rice to the side of the dish and break the eggs into the unfilled space in the container. Sprinkle with 1 teaspoon soy sauce and scramble.
- When eggs are cooked through, mix the eggs into the rice.
- Remove from the heat and stir in the scallions.
- Sprinkle with sesame oil and serve.

45: Wild Cajun Spiced Salmon

Cajun Salmon with a simple natively constructed preparation made with flavors you as of now have in your washroom that can be heated, cooked, dish singed, or barbecued. This solid supper is prepared in under fifteen minutes and comparable to any eatery variant.

Cajun Salmon that is hot, smoky, and prepared right away makes for a simple and solid supper that can be cooked inside or outside on the flame broil. Serve it warm or cold for a protein-stuffed supper that is scrumptious. We likewise make this Blackened Salmon and Brown Sugar Salmon consistently, so add these to your go-to salmon plans.

Ingredients:

- 3 tsp olive oil, separated
- 2 6 oz. filets of salmon
- 2 tbsp. Cajun preparing

- Legitimate salt + broke black pepper, to taste

Method:

- Preheat the stove to 425 degrees C.
- Brush a preparing dish or oven with 1 tsp olive oil.
- Put salmon filets down into dish — skin-side down if they have skin.
- Brush 1 tsp of olive oil over each filet.
- Sprinkle with Kosher salt + broke black pepper.
- Sprinkle each filet with 1 tbsp. of Cajun preparing each, tapping and kneading the flavoring into the filet like a rub.
- Rub onto the sides of the filets too.
- Spot in the broiler and heat for 15 minutes or until filets effectively drop.
- The safe inward temperature for fish is 62.8 °C/145 °F.

This Healthy Beef Stroganoff recipe is outstanding both for what it offers—all the smooth, comfortable kind of the exemplary recipe, eased up with a couple of solid ingredient trades and made simpler in the simmering pot—just as for what it doesn't. This stewing pot meat stroganoff is made without canned soup.

Ingredients:

- 1 tablespoon margarine
- ½ teaspoon salt
- 1 teaspoon arranged mustard
- 2-pound meat hurl cook
- ½ teaspoon ground black pepper
- salt and ground black pepper to taste
- ⅓ cup white wine
- ¼ cup generally useful flour
- ½ pound white mushrooms, cut
- 1 ¼ cups decreased sodium meat stock, separated
- ⅓ cup light acrid cream
- 4 green onions, cut (white and green parts)
- 2 tablespoons spread, partitioned

Method:

- Remove any fat and cartilage from the meal and cut into strips 1/2-inch thick by 2-inches in length.

- Sprinkle with 1/2 teaspoon salt and 1/2 teaspoon pepper.
- Soften 1 tablespoon margarine in a large oven over medium heat.
- Add mushrooms and green onions and cook, mixing once in a while, until mushrooms are sautéed, around 6 minutes.
- Remove to a bowl and add 1 tablespoon margarine to the oven.
- Cook and mix one a large portion of the hamburger strips until caramelized, around 5 minutes, then remove to a bowl.
- Rehash with the excess spread and hamburger strips.
- Empty wine into the hot oven and deglaze the container, scraping up any sautéed bits.
- Join flour and 1/4 cup meat stock in a container with a firmly fitting cover and shake until consolidated.
- Stir into the oven, racing until smooth.
- Stir in the excess stock and mustard, then return the meat to the container.
- Bring to a stew. Cover and stew until the meat are delicate, around 60 minutes.
- Stir in the readied mushrooms and the acrid cream five minutes before serving. Heat momentarily and sprinkle with salt and pepper.

47: Better Potato Nachos

This tasty and solid yam nachos recipe contains 47.9 grams of protein and 6.4 grams of fiber in only one serving. These yam nachos are solid, clean, and effectively made paleo and vegetarian, as well. Solid Potato Nachos is a sound option in contrast to customary nachos. This recipe is not difficult to follow and is kid-accommodating as well. All you need is a yam, black beans, chicken, and conventional nacho ingredients to make this fast, simple, fun recipe that is diabetes agreeable, gluten-free, heart-healthy, and low in sodium.

Ingredients:

- 18oz lean meat mince
- 14oz can Mexican-style tomatoes
- 23oz potatoes, daintily cut
- 1 onion, finely cleaved
- 15oz can gentle stew beans
- olive shower oil
- ½ cup ground fat-free cheddar
- To serve
- 2 spring onions, finely slashed
- ⅓ cup fat-free harsh cream
- slashed fresh coriander

Method:

- Preheat broiler to 375°F. Cook potatoes in bubbling water for 8-10 minutes until somewhat delicate.
- 2Brown mince in a non-stick oven. Add onion. Cook for a couple of moments.
- Add beans and tomatoes.
- Cook for 4-5 minutes.
- Mastermind a large portion of the potatoes in a big ovenproof dish or split between 4 person dishes.
- Shower with a little olive oil.
- Spoon over mince. Orchestrate remaining potatoes up and over.
- Splash with oil. Sprinkle with cheddar.
- Prepare for 25 minutes.
- Present with acrid cream, spring onions, and coriander.

48: Sheet Pan Chicken and Brussel Sprouts

This is a real stove-to-table sheet-container supper brimming with delicate, crunchy Brussels sprouts and firm, lemony chicken. A simple lemon-and-spice compound spread sprinkles both the chicken and fledglings, which are then finished off with slender lemon cuts that become crunchy in the broiler, offering a decent textural component and a splendid sprinkle of shading and flavor. The key is to cut the lemon adjusts nearly paper-flimsy, so they can fresh up and lose their harshness.

Ingredients:

- 4 cups Brussels sprouts, quartered
- ¾ teaspoon salt, separated
- ½ teaspoon ground cumin
- ¾ teaspoon ground pepper, separated
- ½ teaspoon dried thyme
- ½ teaspoon dried thyme
- 2 tablespoons extra-virgin olive oil, separated
- 1 pound yams, cut into 1/2-inch wedges
- 1 ¼ pound boneless, skinless chicken thighs, managed

Method:

- Preheat broiler to 425 degrees F.
- Toss yams with 1 tablespoon oil and 1/4 teaspoon each salt and pepper in a large bowl.
- Spread equitably on a rimmed preparing sheet. Broil for 15 minutes.
- Toss Brussels sprouts with the leftover 1 tablespoon oil and 1/4 teaspoon each salt and pepper in the bowl.
- Stir into the yams on the preparing sheet.
- Sprinkle chicken with cumin, thyme, and the leftover 1/4 teaspoon of each salt and pepper. Spot on top of the vegetables.
- Broil until the chicken is cooked through and the vegetables are delicate, 10 to 15 minutes more.
- Move the chicken to a serving platter. Mix vinegar into the vegetables and present with the chicken.

This salad may help you to remember a cocktail or a wedge salad. Consider well drink trims, like celery, parsley, green olives, anchovies, or bacon, when choosing what else to add to this dish.

Ingredients:

- 2 tbsp. red wine vinegar
- 2 tbsp. olive oil
- 2 tsp. Worcestershire sauce
- 1/2 tsp. Tabasco
- 2 tsp. arranged horseradish pressed dry
- 1/2 tsp. celery seeds
- Kosher salt and pepper
- 2 celery stems, daintily cut
- 1-16-ounce cherry tomatoes, split
- 1/2 little red onion, daintily cut
- 1 little head green-leaf lettuce, leaves torn
- 1/4 c. level leaf parsley, finely cleaved
- 4 little bone-in pork slashes (1 in. thick, about 2¼ lbs. all-out)

Method:

- Heat barbecue to medium-high.
- In a big bowl, whisk together oil, vinegar, Worcestershire sauce, horseradish, Tabasco, celery seeds, and ¼ teaspoon salt. Toss with tomatoes, celery, and onion.

- Sprinkle pork slashes with 1/2 teaspoon each salt and pepper and barbecue until brilliant earthy colored and just cooked through, 5 to 7 minutes for every side.
- Overlay parsley into tomatoes and serve over pork and greens.

50: Slow-Cooker Black Eyed Peas

This Slow Cooked Black Eyed Peas recipe requires only a couple of minutes of prep, then everything gets toss in the sluggish cooker! Black peered toward peas are the ideal solace food. Made with an extra ham bone and stewed in a rich delectable stock, these Slow Cooker Black Eyed Peas and Collard Greens are a tasty expansion to your Fresh Year's Day menu.

Ingredients:

- salt, to taste
- 1 shape chicken bouillon
- 6 cups water
- 1 onion, chopped
- 2 cloves garlic, chopped
- 1 pound dried black peered toward peas, arranged and flushed
- 1 jalapeno Chile, cultivated and crushed
- 1 red ringer pepper, stemmed, cultivated, and chopped
- 1 teaspoon ground black pepper
- 8 ounces chopped ham
- 4 cuts bacon, cleaved
- ½ teaspoon cayenne pepper

- 1 ½ teaspoons cumin

Method:

- Empty the water into a lethargic cooker, add the bouillon block, and mix to break down.
- Join the black peered toward peas, onion, salt, Chile pepper, garlic, jalapeno pepper, bacon, cayenne pepper, ham, cumin, and pepper; mix to mix.
- Cover the lethargic cooker and cook on Low for 6 to 8 hours until the beans are delicate.

51: Salmon and Veggies at 5:30 P.M.

Barbecued salmon and veggies make for a beautiful and adjusted fish supper that is prepared in only minutes. The flame broil turns the salmon flaky and sodden while softening the fresh pepper and onion pieces. Balance the supper with earthy-colored rice or quinoa. This carb-cognizant dinner is loaded with protein and nutrients. Transform it into a sheet oven supper recipe if you don't have a meal dish.

Ingredients:

- salt, to taste
- pepper, to taste
- 4 cloves garlic, crushed
- 2 teaspoons ginger
- 4 tablespoons olive oil
- 4 tablespoons lemon juice
- 2 tablespoons fresh thyme
- 2 salmon filets

- 2 lb. little red potato (910 g), or yellow, quartered
- 1 package asparagus, about 1 pound (455g)

Method:

- Preheat the stove to 400°F (200°C).
- Cover a sheet dish with foil or material paper. Spread out potatoes in the oven and sprinkle with olive oil. Sprinkle with salt, pepper, 2 cloves of garlic, and 1 tablespoon lemon juice.
- Heat for 30 minutes.
- Make salmon coating.
- Join salt, pepper, 2 garlic cloves, 1 tablespoon thyme, ginger, 2 tablespoons of olive oil, and 2 tablespoons of lemon juice. Blend well.
- Remove potatoes from the broiler and push them to the top or side of your oven.
- Spot your salmon filets on the container.
- Brush the two sides of the salmon with the coating.
- Spot asparagus on the dish and top with 1 tablespoon olive oil, salt, 1 tablespoon lemon squeeze, and pepper.
- Sprinkle 1 tsp of thyme on the potatoes and asparagus.
- Prepare for 10-12 minutes. (The salmon should piece effectively with a fork when it's prepared.) Enjoy!

52: Poached Egg with Asparagus and Tomato

This supper is a fast and simple path for any recipe phobe to prepare an overly scrumptious dish in a matter of moments. With their various medical advantages, eggs are extraordinary at any time and taste scrumptious when presented with fresh asparagus lances.

Ingredients:

- 1 tablespoon honey
- 1 tablespoon Dijon mustard
- 2 shallots, shaved slight
- ½ cup olive oil
- 1 lemon, supreme, and juiced*
- Coarse salt and fresh broke pepper, to taste
- 2 garlic cloves, crushed
- 2 packages asparagus, bottoms managed
- 4 Creole tomatoes, cut in thick adjusts
- 6 tablespoons parmesan, ground
- 4 eggs

Method:

- Carry a big pot of salted water to stew and keep prepared.
- In the mixing bowl, add Dijon mustard, shallots, honey, lemon Supremes, and juice. Race in olive oil and sprinkle with salt and pepper. Put dressing in a safe spot.
- In the large oven, add a sprinkle of olive oil and singe asparagus stems in clumps with a spot of crushed garlic. Sprinkle with salt and pepper.
- Spot stems in a single layer in the oven so they don't steam and overcook.

- If planning early, place promptly into the cooler, serve chilled.
- Have everything plated and all set before poaching eggs, as they are time-touchy.
- On large plates mastermind cuts of tomato, marginally covering one another.
- Shower tomatoes with olive oil and sprinkle with salt and pepper.
- Gap and organize singed asparagus on plates.
- To poach eggs, add a sprinkle of white vinegar to a pot of stewing water.
- Whirl spoon around in your water to make it move in roundabout movement and afterward break and drop your eggs into the center.
- Delicately twirl water.
- Poach 2-4 minutes to cook, or until whites are firm to contact and focus are giggly.
- To gather, place one poached egg on top of each heap of asparagus.
- Blend vinaigrette and delicately spoon over the egg, asparagus, and tomatoes.
- Get done with freshly ground parmesan and serve right away.

53: Yogurt with Blueberries

A simple blend of Greek yogurt and blueberries gets an additional dash of pleasantness from brilliant honey. It's the ideal equilibrium of protein and fiber to keep you empowered. These two food varieties draw out the best in one another.

The high fiber substance of the berries (just about four grams for every cup) reinforces the sound microbes found in yogurt, also known as probiotics, assisting it with enduring the dangerous excursion through the stomach-related lot. Once in the gut, the probiotics assist the body with engrossing the solvent fiber of the blueberries.

Ingredients:

- ¼ cup blueberries
- 1 cup nonfat plain Greek yogurt

Method:

- Spot yogurt in a bowl and top with blueberries.

54: Feta and Tomato Omelets

Add the Mediterranean contort to your plate with this Feta and Tomato Omelets recipe with feta cheddar, black olives, and tomato. Greek omelet is an exceptionally flexible dish one can appreciate at any time. It very well may be filled in as a filling high-energy breakfast, a quick bite with some dry town bread, or even dinner.

This Feta and Tomato Omelets recipe is truly simple to plan and incorporates basic ingredients, however, the taste is truly flawless and fresh. You will adore the blend of feta and tomato.

Ingredients:

- 3 black Kalamata olives
- 1/2 tomato, slashed into shapes
- 60g/2 oz. feta cheddar disintegrated
- 2 tbsps. olive oil
- a squeeze dried oregano
- 3 large eggs
- ground Graviera cheddar to decorate
- salt and freshly ground pepper

Method:

- To make this heavenly Greek omelet recipe start by setting up the ingredients first.
- Remove the seeds and add juice from the tomato and cut the tissue into little 3D squares. Put in a safe spot.

- Remove the pits from the olives and cut them into little pieces. Put in a safe spot.
- Disintegrate the feta cheddar with your hands or utilizing a fork and set it aside.
- Break the eggs in a bowl and sprinkle with salt and pepper. Beat the eggs with a fork until consolidated.
- Heat a little medium nonstick griddle over medium heat.
- Add 2 tbsps. olive oil and the beaten eggs. Utilizing a spatula, drag the omelet towards the one finish of the oven and slant the dish to allow the crude eggs to fill the unfilled side.
- Rehash this interaction for approx. 1-2 minutes until the omelet is cooked. (the eggs are set yet the top is still marginally clammy)
- Remove the dish from the heat and add the tomato, feta cheddar, olives, oregano.
- Slip the spatula under the omelet, tip to release, and delicately overlay the omelet fifty-fifty.
- Sprinkle with ground cheddar and serve.

55: Spicy Chocolate Keto Fat Bombs

Keto chocolate is high in fat and sugar-free for a low carb contort, however all you'll taste is smooth, velvety dull chocolate flavor combined with an impactful zest blend that makes certain to warm you up a bit! It's so natural to make chocolate at home with only a couple of ingredients.

Try it and see with your own eyes. These scrumptious and delish keto fat bombs make certain to be hit. Fill in as keto pastries, keto snacks, keto sweet treat, or make to take to parties. These are even raved about by people who don't follow a ketogenic diet/lifestyle.

You can add a wide range of additional ingredients to the focal point of the hot cocoa bombs, sprinkles to the outside, or considerably more dissolved chocolate. They look so extravagant and beautiful, so normally, they are stunning endowments as well.

Ingredients:

- ⅓ cup cocoa powder
- ½ cup sugar
- ⅓ cup weighty cream powder
- 7 oz. ChocZero sugar free chocolate chips (1 sack of milk or dim chips)

Optional:

- sugar free sprinkles
- 1 tsp coconut oil
- ¼ cup ChocZero without sugar white chocolate chips

Method:

- Microwave the sugar free chocolate chips for 30 seconds.
- Mix. If they aren't softened microwave at 15 seconds spans, mixing after each.
- When they are about 75% softened simply mix until they are liquefied.

- Spoon a stacking teaspoon into every cavity of a 2-inch circle form. Utilize the rear of the teaspoon to push the chocolate up the edges.
- As it sets keep pushing chocolate up the sides to make a thicker shell.
- Spot a storing tablespoon of the hot cocoa blend inside a large portion of the circles.
- Spoon on dissolved chocolate around the edge.
- Top with the second 50% of the circle.
- Optional: Drizzle with extra liquefied chocolate blended in with 1 teaspoon of coconut oil and top with sprinkles.
- Refrigerate until fixed.
- Spot a hot cocoa bomb into a mug.
- Pour 6-ounce of hot milk on chocolate bomb.
- Mix until smooth.

Chapter#5

Breakfast

56: Baked Egg with Ham and Spinach

Heated Egg with Ham and Spinach plans permit you to appreciate a nutritious meal when you're in a hurry. Their little, biscuit estimated extents also make them the ideal menu thing for evening snacks, picnics, or social affairs. If you have a bunch of demanding eaters on your hands, these simple spinach and ham egg heats give a fun, reduced-down food even kids will appreciate. Look at our simple spinach and ham egg prepares recipe below to begin.

Ingredients:

- 100g baby spinach leaves
- 15g spread, extra to oil
- 100ml cream
- 4 big eggs
- Ocean salt and freshly ground black pepper
- 25g goat's cheddar

- Buttered sourdough toast fingers, to serve
- 100g hand-cut cooked ham, finely chopped

Method:

- Preheat the stove to 180°C/350°F/Gas mark 4.
- Heat the spread in a little oven and rapidly sauté the spinach until withered.
- Season to taste and deplete off any overabundance fluid.
- Spread 4 profound ramekins and spoon a little hill of spinach in the lower part of everyone, then disperse over the ham and goat's cheddar.
- Break an egg and season with salt, then add a fourth of the cream to every ramekin.
- Mastermind the ramekins in a broiling tin and pour in sufficient bubbling water to come mostly up every ramekin.
- Spot in the oven and heat for 15 minutes, until the eggs are simply set yet the yolks are as yet runny.
- Set a ramekin on a warmed plate and add sourdough toast fingers to serve.

57: Lighter Baked Mushrooms

These mushrooms are heated in a delicious prepared cream sauce and they're wonderful as a gathering hors d'oeuvre or as a side dish for breakfast. They might be The Best Baked Mushrooms I've at any point had. These prepared mushrooms are too easy to make and they're flavorful.

Ingredients:

- 1 tsp olive oil
- 1 stick celery, daintily cut
- 30g/1oz baby spinach
- 1 tomato, split
- 1 spring onion, daintily cut
- salt and freshly ground black pepper
- 20g/¾oz fresh breadcrumbs
- 1 bacon emblem (30g/1oz), generally chopped
- 2 big, level Portobello mushrooms (150g/5½oz complete weight), cleaned off, stalks finely chopped

Method:

- Preheat the stove to 220C/200C Fan/Gas 7.
- Heat the oil in a little griddle over medium heat.
- Add the mushroom stems, spring onion, celery, and bacon and cook for 1–2 minutes, or until mellowed.
- Stir in the breadcrumbs and spinach and season.
- Spot the mushrooms cup-side up on a preparing plate.
- Season the tomato and spot it on the preparing plate.

- Spoon the filling into the mushrooms and heat for 10–15 minutes, or until they have mellowed.
- Serve the mushrooms with the tomato.

58: Banana and Coconut Porridge

Utilizing bananas is the best way to tenderly improve. The banana essentially softens (with a little assistance from your spoon during the cooking time frame) into the entire thing, giving a lovely imbuement of supporting pleasantness. In this recipe, I'll be telling you the best way to make an excessively simple porridge.

Ingredients:

- 50g (½ cup) oats
- 350ml approx. (1 ½ cup) water
- 1 ready banana (medium measured)
- Sprinkle maple syrup
- 1 tablespoon slashed creamed coconut

Method:

- Add the oats to a little oven (without top).
- Cleave the banana into slices.
- Add ¾ of the water to the dish and switch on the heat.
- The cooking period will associate with 15 minutes.
- Carry the substance to the reduce and afterward go down to a stew.
- Stir incidentally during this time.
- If the water begins to dry out excessively fast essentially add somewhat more water as required.

(Water sum will fluctuate from one bunch to another and contingent upon what amount is being steamed off).

- Press in the cut banana as it cooks, with your spoon, until in the long run it 'dissolves into the entire porridge.
- Take a little measure of the creamed coconut and cleave finely.
- If it's not too much trouble, note: creamed coconut arrives in a strong square structure and melts after warming, making it a fantastic thickening specialist and flavor for this dish.

59: Banana Smoothie

This solid banana smoothie is basic and loaded with protein, fiber, and potassium. Mix it up this week for a solid smoothie breakfast or tidbit. Bananas are an extraordinary decision for making custom-made smoothies. Use them as a base and add various fruits for a speedy and simple mixed beverage.

Ingredients:

- 4 ice 3D shapes
- 1 banana
- 2 cups skim or decreased fat milk
- 1 tablespoon decreased fat plain yogurt
- ½ teaspoon cinnamon

Method:

- Spot all ingredients in blender and cycle until smooth
- Fill two glasses and serve right away.

60: Toast with Ham and Cheese

I can hardly wait to share my number one ham and cheddar sandwich recipe, yet before I do, I have parcels to enlighten you regarding this simple meal. All the data I got some answers concerning a simple ham and cheddar sandwich were insane jeans.

Ingredients:

- Dijon mustard
- 4 liberal slices of ham
- 8 toast slices of bread
- 80g Edam delectable cheddar, cut
- 2/3 cup milk
- 50g spread
- salt and freshly ground black pepper
- 3 Henergy Cage Free eggs

Method:

- Orchestrate 4 of the bread slices on a board and top with ham and cheddar.
- Spread the leftover bread slices with a little Dijon mustard.
- Make a sandwich with the mustard looking into the sandwich.
- Whisk the milk and eggs together.
- Season with salt and fresh black pepper.
- Heat a big oven or grill hot plate to medium heat.

- If it is too hot and the bread will consume before the cheddar dissolves.
- Empty the egg blend into a shallow dish and sit one sandwich in the fluid, turning over after around 20 seconds.
- Dissolve a little margarine in the griddle or hot plate and cook the sandwiches in clumps (absorbing each egg combination first) until brilliant on the two sides and the cheddar has softened.
- Serve hot!

61: Yogurt and Muesli

These solid yogurt and muesli breakfast cups don't simply look pretty they are scrumptious as well. Layers of velvety yogurt, toasted muesli, and fresh berries. Simple ingredients to stir your taste buds. Ideal for breakfast, morning tea, or a solid bite.

Ingredients:

- 1 cup Greek-style yogurt
- 1 cup toasted muesli
- 2 tsp strawberry jam
- ½ cup fresh berries

Method:

- Gap half of the muesli into the lower part of the 2 cups or containers.
- Next split part of the Greek yogurt between the cups and top for certain berries.

- Rehash with residual muesli and Greek yogurt.
- Ladle 1tsp of strawberry jam on every cup.
- Separation the leftover berries over the top.

62: Porridge Oats with Apricot Compote

This simple oats recipe cooks in only 5 minutes. While this solid oats recipe calls for coconut and apricots, other dried fruits, like raisins and cranberries, likewise are delectable.

Ingredients:

- 1 cup water
- ½ teaspoon ground cinnamon
- ½ cup antiquated moved oats
- 6 dried apricots, chopped
- 1 tablespoon unsweetened smashed coconut

Method:

- Consolidate oats, water, and cinnamon in a little pan.
- Heat to the point of boiling over high heat.
- Reduce heat to a stew and cook, blending periodically, until smooth, around 5 minutes.
- Serve finished off with apricots and coconut.

63: Apple and Cinnamon Breakfast Pot

Apple Cinnamon Overnight Oats make a thick, rich, and simple breakfast choice when mornings get going. Make this recipe the prior night for a yummy meal with warm flavors and sweet apples.

Ingredients:

- run of cinnamon
- 1/3 cup quinoa, cooked
- 1/4 cup almond milk
- 2 tablespoons coconut milk yogurt
- 1/4 cup bounces red plant gluten-free cereal
- 1/3 cup meagerly cut apple
- 1 tablespoon sugar-coated walnuts, squashed
- 1 tablespoon pomegranate arils
- a sprinkle of nectar (or maple syrup for veggie lover)

Method:

- To a little bowl add gluten-free oats and almond milk.
- Mix to blend.
- Spot in the microwave, uncovered, and cook for 1-2 minutes.
- Until wanted consistency.

- Eliminate from the microwave and add cooked quinoa, cut apples, coconut milk yogurt, pomegranate arils, sugar-coated walnuts, and a scramble of cinnamon.
- Shower with nectar (or maple syrup for vegetarian).
- Serve.

64: Toast with Mashed Banana and Yogurt

Yogurt is an incredible element for adding to banana bread and other heated products. It keeps the bread wet, delicate, and very tasty without utilizing a big load of margarine or oil. You'll need to utilize plain yogurt for this recipe, not pre-improved. I have not tried Greek-style yogurt in this recipe, however would figure that it would make a somewhat denser part since it has less dampness than customary yogurt.

Ingredients:

- 2 big eggs
- 1/2 tsp heating pop
- 1/4 tsp ocean salt
- 1/4 cup (60 ml) maple syrup
- 1/4 cup (50 g) earthy colored sugar
- 1/2 cups (180 g) universally handy flour
- 2 medium-sized ready bananas (200 g or 1 cup squashed)
- 1/2 cup (115 g) plain or vanilla Greek yogurt
- Optional add-ins: 1/2 cup chocolate chips/raisins/nuts

Method:

- Preheat your oven to 350°F (176°C), and softly oil a 9 x 5 (23cm x 13cm) part dish.

- In a big blending bowl, join the flour, preparing pop, and salt. Put in a safe spot.
- In a more modest blending bowl, gently beat the eggs until the yolks fall to pieces.
- Speed in the pounded bananas, yogurt, maple syrup, and sugar (if utilizing), blending until smooth.
- Add the wet ingredients to the dry ingredients, blending delicately until just joined. Don't overmix.
- In case you're adding any blend-ins, overlay them in at this point.
- Empty the player into the part oven, spreading it out equally, and prepare for 40-45 minutes, or until a toothpick embedded into the center confesses all.
- Eliminate the bread from the oven and let it cool in the search for gold for 10 minutes before moving it to a cooling rack to cool totally.

65: Poached Egg On Toast

Eggs are a high wellspring of protein and make a solid breakfast. With an assortment of egg plans accessible to us, one delectable American egg recipe is poached eggs with toast. Made with the integrity of eggs, spread, vinegar, and toasted bread this morning meal recipe will get one of your top choices. This easy-to-make recipe is ideal for the ones who need to treat themselves with a lip-smacking and sound breakfast to begin their day on the correct note.

Ingredients:

- Eggs big
- Buttered wholemeal toast
- 2 – 3 glugs of white refined vinegar about a tablespoon

Method:

- Fill a griddle with 3.5cm of bubbling water from the pot (energy productive).
- Add the vinegar and take it back to the bubble.
- Break the egg into a ramekin/little bowl and delicately bring down the egg into the water tipping out tenderly, proceed with the number of eggs required.
- Time the eggs for 3 minutes. If you incline toward yours firmer simply increase the time by a moment.
- Utilizing an opened spoon, place your eggs on several sheets of kitchen move to smear away any leftover water.

- Spot on buttered toast and present with a sprinkle of salt or ketchup whenever wanted.

66: Wheat Cereal with Banana and Raisins

Delightfully made oat that can help stimulate the beginning of your day. This crunchy, exemplary grain is made with fresh, toasted wheat chips offset with the satisfyingly sweet taste of genuine banana pieces blended right in. Similarly, however nutritious as it seems to be delectable, this grain gives a decent wellspring of six fundamental nutrients and minerals so you can kick your free day off right.

Ingredients:

- 1 egg
- 1/4 cups flour
- 1/4 tsp. salt
- 1 Tbsp. heating powder
- 1 cup smashed wheat cereal
- 1 cup fat-free milk
- 2 Tbsp. margarine
- 1/2 cup raisins
- 1 cup pounded ready banana (2 big)
- 1/3 cup solidly pressed earthy colored sugar

Method:

- Preheat stove to 400 degrees.
- Blend flour, preparing powder, and salt in a big bowl.

- Blend grain and milk in another big bowl; let stand 5 minutes.
- Stir in egg, banana, sugar, and margarine.
- Add to the flour blend; mix just until soaked (hitter will be uneven).
- Stir in raisins.
- Spoon player into a biscuit container, which has been splashed with a no-stick cooking shower, and fill each cup 66% full.
- Heat 20 minutes or until brilliant earthy colored.
- Serve warm.

67: Fried Eggs with Smoked Salmon

Smoked salmon can be bought in two structures: Hot smoked and cold smoked. Hot smoked salmon is in a real sense cooked during the smoked interaction, which makes it firm and pungent. Cold smoked salmon isn't cooked, and it has a fragile and rich surface. Fried eggs are not difficult to make as long as you observe a couple of rules.

Ingredients:

- 6 eggs
- 75ml milk
- 1 tbsp. margarine
- 4 slices bread, like brioche or sourdough
- 4 spring onions, washed and meagerly cut
- 1 x 100g pack smoked salmon
- little bundle fresh chives, slashed

Method:

- Break the eggs into a big container or blending bowl. Add the milk and a little flavoring, then race until light yellow – the children will cherish assisting with this part.
- Stir in a large part of the chives.

- Dissolve the spread in a griddle set over medium heat. Add the spring onions and fry for 3-4 minutes, until mollified.
- Turn up the heat somewhat and add the beaten egg. Leave it to cook for 20 seconds, then tenderly blend it in with a spatula, or wooden spoon. Cook for an additional 20 seconds and afterward blend once more. Rehash until cooked through.
- In the meantime, toast the bread and request that the children spread it. Cut into triangles and mastermind 2 on each plate.
- To serve, split the eggs between the 4 plates. The children would then be able to finish off with the smoked salmon and remaining chives.

68: Healthy Berry Banana Smoothie

The Berry Banana Smoothie is plentiful in potassium and nutrient C. This recipe also has yogurt in it, which gives it regular probiotics, fundamental for processing. Berry Smoothies give you more fiber and supplements than normal juices, assisting you with remaining appropriately hydrated while supporting your safe framework. You can likewise substitute red, yellow raspberries, or even blueberries. I've attempted grapes, don't go there, it's yucky.

Ingredients:

- 1 Banana
- 10 blackberries
- 8 Strawberries
- 1/2 Cup Odwalla's Orange Juice
- 1/2 cup vanilla yogurt

Method:

- Join all ingredients together in a blender and puree until smooth.

69: Blackberry and Apple Crumble Smoothie

In case you're searching for something sweet, utilize more agave honey. I simply use contact since I would not like to detract from the kinds of blackberries and apples.

Ingredients:

- 1 apple, cored and cut
- 300g/10½oz frozen blended berries
- 200ml/7floz semi-skimmed milk
- 25g/1oz porridge oats, with additional fiber
- 150g/5½oz without fat common yogurt
- 10g/¼oz chopped almonds

Method:

- Spot the berries, apples, milk, yogurt, oats, and nuts in a blender and mix until smooth.
- Add cold water, a little at a time, to achieve a smooth consistency and mix once more.
- Fill glasses and serve.

Chapter#6: Lunch

70: Beetroot, Green Bean and Feta Salad

This is a dazzling stormy salad of beetroot, green beans, and goat's cheddar, dressed with a squeezed orange, shallot, and mustard dressing. The tones are lovely and it would make a beautiful starter or even a principal course salad. Green beans are a cell reinforcement genius. They contain a variety of carotenoids and flavonoids which have all been appeared to have health properties.

Ingredients:

- 1tbsp white wine vinegar
- 2tbsp extra virgin olive oil
- 1tsp Dijon mustard
- 1 shallot, finely slashed
- Zing and fragments 1 big orange
- 100g baby spinach leaves
- 250g pack Extra Special Extra Fine Beans

- 100g frozen expansive beans, defrosted and shelled
- 1 medium carrot, ground
- 2 cooked beetroots, chopped
- 2tbsp toasted hazelnuts, generally slashed
- 100g Chosen by you Greek Feta, disintegrated
- Dry bread, to serve

Method:

- Put the oil, vinegar, mustard, orange zing, and shallot in a bowl. Race with a fork.
- In a big bowl, blend the orange fragments, fine beans, spinach, wide beans, carrot, and beetroot. Pour over the dressing and throw it together.
- Top with the feta and hazelnuts.
- Serve rightly with dry bread.

71: Lentil, Cherry Tomato, and Feta Salad

Take your taste buds to the reviving kinds of the Mediterranean with each chomp of this stunning Greek lentil salad recipe. A totally delightful and very sound Greek-style lentil salad with feta cheddar and fresh vegetables. Overflowing with fresh and energetic tones and flavors, regardless of whether eaten as a tidbit, side, or light vegan dinner, this very simple feta lentil salad recipe never disappoints!

Ingredients:

- 1/2 Tbsp. (20 mL) red wine vinegar
- 1/4 cups (310 mL) entire green lentils
- Kosher salt
- 1 garlic clove, ground or minced
- 3 tbsp. (45 mL) olive oil
- fresh ground black pepper
- 3 tbsp. (45 mL) chopped dill, in addition to extra for sprinkling
- 3 tbsp. (45 mL) chopped chives, in addition to extra for sprinkling
- 3 tbsp. (45 mL) chopped Italian parsley, in addition to extra for sprinkling
- 3 oz. (90 g) Feta cheddar disintegrated

- 1/2 lb. (250 g), cherry tomatoes, split or quartered assuming huge
- flaky ocean salt, for sprinkling
- 1 torpedo onion, managed and daintily cut (or use a little red onion or two shallots)

Method:

- Add the onion to a medium bowl, and throw with vinegar and a touch of Kosher salt. Let sit while you set up the lentils.
- Spot lentils in a medium pot filled 2/3's with water, and heat to the point of boiling over medium-high heat, mixing every so often.
- Lessen heat to medium-low, and stew until the lentils are simply delicate (around 15 minutes).
- Begin checking for doneness around 13 to 14 minutes, since, supposing that you overcook the lentils, they will go to mush.
- Channel the lentils well, then throw with the marinated onion.
- Stir in olive oil and garlic, and season to taste with salt and pepper.
- Allow lentils to cool totally.
- Add slashed spices to the bowl alongside half of the tomatoes and feta, throwing to consolidate.
- Pour salad onto a serving platter, then top with residual tomatoes and feta.
- Get done with a sprinkling of spices, flaky ocean salt, and ground black pepper.

72: Chicken Tikka Salad

This chicken salad is an extraordinary expansion of your week-by-week supper revolution. It's loaded with chickpeas, marinated chicken breast, and sprinkled with a delicious yogurt blend. This speedy chicken tikka salad is stacked with fresh veggies, chickpeas, and delicious marinated chicken, for a simple, light lunch.

Ingredients:

- Red stew glue 1/2 teaspoons
- Thick yogurt 4 tablespoons
- Ginger-garlic glue 2 teaspoons
- Garam masala powder 1/2 teaspoon
- Almonds whitened and stripped 1 tablespoon
- Salt to taste
- Juice of ½ lemon
- Spring onion bulb 1
- Oil for barbecuing
- Fresh basil leaves 6-7
- Ice sheet lettuce leaves 4-5
- Fresh mint leaves 15-20
- Lollo rosso lettuce leaves 6-7
- Mustard glue 2 teaspoons

For Dressing:

- Tomato juice 1/3 cup
- Balsamic vinegar 1 teaspoon
- Olive oil 1 tablespoon

- Salt to taste
- Squashed black peppercorns to taste
- Boneless Chicken cut into little pieces 500 grams

Method:

- Take yogurt in a bowl. Add red stew glue and ginger-garlic glue.
- Toast almonds till delicately sautéed.
- Add salt, garam masala powder, and lemon juice to the yogurt and blend well. Add chicken pieces and blend well. Put to the side to marinate for 4 hours.
- Move toasted almonds to another bowl and cool to room temperature.
- Heat some oil in a non-stick flame broil container. Spot marinated chicken pieces on it and barbecue till the chicken is completely cooked.
- To make the salad, corner to corner cut spring onion bulb and spot in a bowl. Generally, cleave basil leaves and add them along with mint leaves.
- Tear Iceberg and lollo rosso lettuce leave and add.
- To make the dressing, take tomato juice in a bowl.
- Add mustard glue, Balsamic vinegar, salt, olive oil, and squashed peppercorns and blend well.
- Reduce chicken tikka from heat and cut further into more modest pieces.
- Add dressing and a part of the chicken pieces to the salad and throw well.

- Move the salad on a serving plate, decorate with staying chicken pieces and toasted almonds, and serve right away.

73: Tuna and Bean Salad

This is a pillar in my home, something you can generally put together for a simple quick bite. The true form would call for fish pressed in olive oil, yet I lean toward water-stuffed fish. The salad packs a ton of protein, from the beans, yet also from the fish, which is likewise a superb wellspring of Omega-3 unsaturated fats. This simple, across-the-board feast, a fish salad is made with straightforward ingredients and washroom staples to make a lunch that is fresh and filling.

Ingredients:

- 15-ounce cannellini beans, flushed and depleted (or Great Northern beans)
- 4 cups arugula (or spinach or other most loved lettuce)
- 5-ounce white tuna fish pressed in water, depleted
- 1/4 cup cut olives (green, Kalamata, or your number one assortment)
- 1/2 cup cherry tomatoes, divided
- Meagerly cut red onion
- 1/2 lemon
- 1/4 cup disintegrated feta cheddar
- 2 tablespoons extra virgin olive oil
- Fit salt and fresh ground black pepper

Method:

- In a big bowl or two more modest dishes, consolidate the arugula, white beans, fish, tomatoes, olives, and red onion.
- Sprinkle with the olive oil and the juice from the lemon. Throw to join.
- Top with disintegrated feta cheddar and season to taste with fit salt and black pepper.

74: Prawns with Cauliflower Curry

Low-fat and high-protein prawns pair superbly with fresh salsa and cauliflower couscous. Prawns are regularly clear when crude yet get their particular pink or red tone on being cooked. a single word of alert – if purchasing unpeeled prawns, smell for freshness, and search for brilliant, glossy shells that make them spring left in them.

Ingredients:

- Cauliflower isolated into medium florets 1 little
- Tiger prawns shelled and deveined 500 grams
- Sugar 1 teaspoon
- Salt to taste
- Juice of 1 lemon
- Oil 1 tablespoon
- Garlic cloves finely chopped 2
- Squashed black peppercorns 1/2 teaspoon
- Onion finely chopped 1 medium
- 10,000-foot chilies finely cleaved 2
- Star anise broiled and powdered 1
- Coconut milk 2 cups
- Fresh coriander leaves finely chopped 1/2 tablespoon
- Fenugreek seeds (methi dana) broiled and powdered 1 teaspoon

Method:

- Put prawns in a bowl, add lemon squeeze and salt, blend well, and put in a safe spot for fifteen minutes.

- Heat oil in a non-stick wok, add onion, garlic, and chilies, and sauté for three to four minutes.
- Add cauliflower and blend and cook for a few minutes.
- Add sugar, powdered star anise, and powdered fenugreek seeds and blend well.
- Add coconut milk and blend once more.
- Decrease heat and cook for ten to fifteen minutes.
- Add marinated prawns and cook till the prawns are finished.
- Add salt, squashed peppercorns, and coriander leaves.
- Blend and stew briefly. Move the curry into a serving bowl and serve hot.

75: Fish and Red Pepper Sandwich

You can do such countless things in a sandwich. This recipe is only one of my numerous varieties of fish sandwiches. It's somewhat sweet from the simmered red pepper, however has a peppery nibble from the watercress. If you don't have watercress, don't stress, use arugula! Try not to have arugula? Use some baby spinach and simply add an extra touch of pepper into your fish combination. This recipe is a scrumptious sandwich to welcome on a cookout.

Ingredients:

- ¼ cup slashed fresh basil leaves
- 1 tablespoon extra-virgin olive oil
- 2 6-ounce jars of fish pressed in water (depleted)
- ¼ teaspoon black pepper
- ⅓ cup bumped broiled red peppers, daintily cut
- 1 teaspoon red wine vinegar

Method:

- In a medium bowl, put basil leaves, consolidate the fish, pepper, olive oil, and vinegar.
- Spread the combination on your favorite bread or roll.

76: Fish Fingers with Tomato Salsa

Another best recipe for your lunch is Fish Fingers with Tomato Salsa. This is a simple to make a recipe that many people love everywhere in the world. I will share every one of the ingredients and making methods for this recipe. You can without much of a stretch make it at your home.

Ingredients:

- 4 eggs
- 1 cup flour
- 2 tbsp. spread
- 3 potatoes, stripped
- Vegetable oil, to broil
- Salt and black pepper
- 1 onion, finely cleaved
- 170 g tin fish
- Small bunch parsley, cleaved
- 155 g tin pilchards
- 1 cup breadcrumbs

Method:

- Preheat stove to 180°C.
- Heat the potatoes until delicate, then squash with the spread until smooth.
- Heat 2 tbsp. oil, fry the onion with pepper and salt for 5 minutes.

- Channel the fish. Wash the pilchards well and chip them into pieces.
- Blend squashed potato, fish, onion, pilchards, parsley, 2 eggs, and ½ cup flour.
- Spot the leftover flour, 2 whisked eggs, and breadcrumbs in 3 dishes.
- Shape the fish blend into fingers and plunge into each bowl thus.
- Light fry the fish fingers for 2 minutes (on both sides).
- Orchestrate the fish fingers on a heating plate and prepare for 15 minutes.

77: Lentil and Tomato Soup

Regardless of whether you're hoping to ease up your dinners or warm up with a steaming bowl of soup, this solid lentil soup recipe is for you! It's one of my unsurpassed top picks and I trust it turns into a staple in your kitchen also.

This soup sort of tastes like a conventional vegetable soup, however with a somewhat more tomato-y stock, in addition to a little grittiness from the lentils. It's overly generous and soothing, which is by and large what I love about a decent bowl of soup in the colder time of year.

Ingredients:

- 3 carrots
- 1 yellow onion
- 2 Tbsp. olive oil
- 2 cloves garlic
- 1 chestnut potato (around 1 lb.)
- 2 15oz. jars stewed tomatoes
- 2 Tbsp. tomato glue
- 1 cup earthy colored lentils
- ½ tsp dried basil
- ½ tsp dried oregano
- ½ tsp paprika
- 4 cups vegetable stock
- 2 Tbsp. soy sauce
- ¼ tsp fresh broke black pepper

Method:

- Mince the garlic, dice the onion, cut the carrots.
- Add the onion, garlic, carrots, and olive oil to a big soup pot and sauté over medium heat until the onions are delicate.
- While the vegetables are cooking, strip and dice the potato into ½-inch shapes.
- Add the tomato glue and proceed to sauté for 2-3 minutes, or until the tomato glue starts to cover the lower part of the pot.
- Add the cubed potato, stewed tomatoes (with juices), paprika, lentils, basil, oregano, pepper, and vegetable stock to the pot.
- Mix to consolidate.
- Spot a cover on top and permit the soup to come up to a bubble.
- When bubbling, turn the heat down to low and allow the soup to stew for around 40 minutes or until the lentils are overly delicate and have started to separate marginally (this thickens the soup).
- Add the soy sauce to the soup, then give it a taste and change the salt if necessary (the aggregate sum will rely upon the salt substance of your vegetable stock).
- Serve hot with dry bread for plunging.

78: Lighter Creamy Mushrooms On Toast

Velvety Mushrooms on Toast is a speedy and simple breakfast or lunch choice that feels undeniably more liberal than it is. A heavenly veggie-lover breakfast, that is not difficult to make vegetarian as well. Stout mushrooms in a smooth and messy sauce, stacked on a thick cut of sourdough toast with a sprinkling of fresh spices.

Ingredients:

- 25 g spread
- 1 tablespoon olive oil
- ½ teaspoon fresh chopped thyme
- Sprinkle of sherry or white wine
- 1 tablespoon fresh cleaved parsley
- 6 tablespoons crème fraiche
- Salt and pepper to taste
- 4 thick cuts bread – toasted (handcrafted bread if conceivable)
- 350 g thickly cut mushrooms (I used chestnut mushrooms)

Method:

- Add the garlic and thyme to the dish, mix through the mushrooms and cook for a further 2 minutes.

- Add a sprinkle of sherry or white wine and the crème fraiche and mix through while keeping on the heat for one more moment or thereabouts.
- Check for preparing and add somewhat salt and pepper to taste.
- Mix through the fresh parsley and top your toast with the smooth mushrooms.

79: Lighter Pea Soup

This light and scrumptious pea soup isn't the ordinary thick and weighty split pea soup that generally strikes a chord when somebody refers to pea soup. It's speedy and too simple to make, as well. A straightforward pea soup makes an exquisite beginning to a spring feast. It's extremely an extraordinary method to use frozen vegetables when the produce area is looking depressing.

Ingredients:

- 1 onion, chopped
- 2 stems celery, managed and chopped
- 1 tsp. Vanns thyme
- 1 lb. Dried split peas, washed
- ½ tsp. Vanns rosemary
- 3 quarts' chicken stock or water
- Vanns kosher salt, to taste
- 3 medium carrots or 2 huge, stripped and chopped
- 1 vanns bay leaf
- Vanns smoked Spanish paprika, to taste
- 4 cuts bacon, cut transversely into ¼-inch pieces
- Vanns black tellicherry peppercorns, fresh ground, to taste
- 1 leek, white, and light green parts just, cut the long way and afterward across into ¼-inch half moons

Method:

- Heat a huge pot, at least 4 quarts, over medium heat.
- When hot, add the slashed bacon and cook, blending much of the time until bacon is fresh and brilliant and all the fat has been delivered.
- Reduce the bacon pieces from the pot with an opened spoon and save.
- Keeping the pot over medium heat, add the chopped onion and sweat until clear and delicate, around 5 minutes.
- Add the chopped carrot, leeks, celery, thyme, and rosemary, and sauté over medium heat until starting to mollify around 10 minutes.
- Add the thyme and rosemary and sauté until fragrant, around 1 more moments.
- Add the split peas and mix to consolidate with the vegetables, and afterward add the stock or water, the held bacon pieces, narrows leaf, and a good spot of Kosher salt.
- Heat to the point of boiling over high heat, scratching the lower part of the pot to get any seared bacon pieces fused into the soup, and afterward bring down the heat to keep a consistent, low stew.
- Stew for around 60 minutes, or until peas are delicate and delicate.
- When peas are cooked, reduce the pot from heat.
- Reduce the sound leaf and move 2 cups of the soup to the bowl of a blender or a hand blender vessel.

- Permit to cool somewhat, so that any sprinkles that depart aren't burning temperature, and afterward mix until smooth.
- Empty the puree once again into the pot of soup and mix to consolidate.
- Season with genuine salt and ground tellicherry peppercorns to taste.
- Serve sprinkled with smoked Spanish paprika.

80: Lighter Hummus with Vegetable Sticks

This hand-crafted Lighter Hummus with Vegetable Sticks recipe is speedy and simple to make, super-smooth and rich, and tastes so fresh and delightful. Give a launch to your day, attempt this delectable hummus with vegetable sticks effectively at home.

Ingredients:

- 1 level tsp tahini
- ½ lemon, squeeze as it were
- 400g tin chickpeas, depleted
- 150g/5½oz broiled red pepper, depleted
- 1 red pepper, seeds reduced, cut into strips, to serve
- squeeze smoked paprika (optional)
- 1 little carrot, stripped and cut into sticks, to serve
- 100g/3½oz sans fat Greek-style plain yogurt

Method:

- Put the lemon juice, chickpeas, yogurt, simmered red pepper, tahini, and smoked paprika, if utilizing, in a food processor.
- Mix until smooth.
- Move into a bowl and present with the vegetable sticks or store in the refrigerator, covered, for as long as three days.

Chapter#7: Dinner

81: Lighter Stir-Fried Beef with Broccoli and Sweetcorn

Searching for a speedy and simple dinner recipe that you can attempt this evening? If you have 15-20 minutes and a couple of essential ingredients, you're good to go to make this delightful pan-fried food. Picking Your Beef, the costliest and most critical part of any dinner is the meat, so pick yours sharply for this fast and simple dinner recipe. Lean meat is rich in protein and a good source of iron. It's additionally delightful in a pan-fried food with broccoli and sweetcorn.

Ingredients:

- 2 tsp soy sauce
- 1 tsp sesame oil
- 100g/3½oz lean meat, cut into strips
- 150ml/5fl oz. meat stock
- 1 garlic clove, finely cleaved

- 80g/3oz tender stem broccoli, generally cleaved
- 30g/1oz dried egg noodles
- 1 spring onion, daintily cut, to embellish
- 40g/1½oz child sweetcorn, generally cleaved
- 20g/¾oz fresh root ginger, stripped and finely cleaved
- ½ red stew, seeds reduced, finely cleaved

Method:

- Blend the meat, oil, garlic, ginger, and stew and leave to marinate in a shallow dish for 15 minutes.
- Heat a wok or pan, add the meat, and pan-fried food for 3–4 minutes.
- Add the broccoli, sweetcorn, and stock and cook for 5 minutes, adding somewhat more stock if essential.
- Spot the noodles in a pot of water, bring them to the bubble and afterward reduce the heat. Cook for 3 minutes, or until just cooked. Drain well.
- Add the noodles to the hamburger and vegetables, stir in the soy sauce, and topping with the spring onion. Serve.

82: Soy and Mirin Cod with Stir Fry

Wild Alaska black cod or sablefish, is rapidly turning into the fish de jour among top culinary experts. The fish is known for its smooth, smooth flavor, its fragile, graceful surface, and rich oil content. The meat is delicate and delicate and liquefies in your mouth. Given these attributes, black cod fits a variety of cooking strategies and styles.

Ingredients:

- 1 tbsp. mirin
- 2 tsp sunflower oil
- 1 tsp rice vinegar
- ½ red pepper (60g/2¼oz), daintily cut
- 50g/1¾oz mangetout, daintily cut
- 1 tsp toasted sesame seeds
- 1 little carrot (50g/1¾oz), daintily cut
- scarcely any twigs fresh coriander (optional)
- 1 tbsp. soy sauce
- 150g/5½oz cod or haddock filet, boneless

Method:

- Spot the fish in a plastic food pack, add the soy, mirin, and rice vinegar.
- Give it a good shake and refrigerate or freeze until prepared to cook.

- Preheat the barbecue to its most sizzling setting and line a little broiling tin with foil.
- Drain the fish, holding the marinade.
- Put the fish on the foil and barbecue for 5 minutes, or until cooked through.
- In the meantime, heat a little wok or griddle over high heat and add the oil. Add the vegetables and pan-fried food for 30 seconds.
- Add 2 tablespoons water and the held marinade and cook for 1–2 minutes, or until hot through.
- Spot the vegetables on a warm plate and top with the fish.
- Dissipate over the sesame seeds and coriander, if utilizing.

83: Butternut Squash Curry with Cauliflower 'Rice'

Butternut squash is a source of vitamins A and C and dietary fiber, and it has a sweet, nutty taste that is like pumpkin. When ready, it turns progressively profound orange - perfect fall tone and gets better and more extravagant. This Butternut Squash Curry with Cauliflower 'Rice' recipe soup isn't a Chinese style. It contains Thai curry glue which is a sodden mix of ground or beat spices as well as flavors and different flavors. Curry glue is fundamentally known as a significant ingredient in Thai cooking. It makes an ideal starter for any dishes in a virus winter.

For the Cauliflower 'Rice':

- 1 tsp olive oil
- 100g/3½oz cauliflower florets
- salt and freshly ground black pepper

For the Curry:

- 150ml/5fl oz. vegetable stock
- 1 tsp rapeseed oil
- 1 tbsp. curry glue
- 250g/9oz butternut squash, cut into 3D shapes
- 200g/7oz tinned cleaved tomatoes
- 40g/1½oz child spinach washed (frozen is likewise fine)

- 1 little onion (75g/2½oz stripped weight), chopped
- 1 garlic clove, finely slashed

Method:

- To make the cauliflower 'rice', preheat the broiler to 200C/180C Fan/Gas 6.
- Heartbeat the cauliflower in a food processor for 30 seconds, or until finely slashed (it should have a similar surface as couscous).
- Blend in the olive oil and season to taste.
- Disperse the combination onto a heating plate and prepare for 15 minutes.
- To make the curry, heat the rapeseed oil in a little, profound pan.
- Add the onion and cook delicately for 2–3 minutes.
- Add the butternut squash, garlic, and curry glue and cook for 2–3 minutes.
- Add the tomatoes and stock, bring to the bubble, then decrease the heat.
- Cover and stew for 15 minutes, blending sometimes.
- Reduce the top and stew for a further 10 minutes.
- Stir in the baby spinach, then cover and cook until shriveled.
- Season to taste with salt and pepper.

84: Prawns with A Spicy Tomato Sauce and Courgetti

This is another fish recipe that requires a couple of moments to cook. Adjusted from Chinese food these prawns in pureed tomatoes are truly simple to cook and you will require a couple of ingredients. This Prawns in Tomato Sauce recipe is another basic and fast prawns pan sear which you can appreciate whenever.

Ingredients:

- 1 tsp ginger garlic glue
- 6 Nos prawns big
- 1 nos big onion cut
- 2 nos green chilies cut
- 3 tbsp. pureed tomatoes
- 2 tbsp. sugar
- 1 tsp red bean stew powder
- 1/2 cup warm water
- Salt according to taste
- 2 tbsp. cooking oil

Method:

- Wash, Clean, and reduce veins of prawns.
- Cut green chilies and onions into reduced-down pieces. Keep to the side.
- Plan ginger garlic glue by granulating not many garlic cloves and a piece of ginger together. Keep to the side.

- In a container, heat cooking oil.
- When oil is hot adding prawns and pan-fried food.
- When the shade of the prawns goes into red/orange, add ginger garlic glue to the container. Blend well.
- When the ginger-garlic glue transforms into brown include the sauce along with everything else.
- Then add bean stew powder, sugar, and salt.
- Blend well.
- Include warm water along with the blend until you get the ideal consistency.
- Include onion and green bean stew along with everything else.
- Stew in low fire for another 1-2 minutes until all consolidate well.
- Check the taste and change salt is vital.
- A tasty prawn dish in pureed tomatoes is prepared to present with singed rice.

85: Lighter Egg Fried Rice

Generally, egg singed rice is a dish intended to go through left-overs - you wouldn't concoct a bunch of fresh rice just to make it, for example. In Asian families, it's very ordinary to have the rice cooker in steady use, so there is in every case warm rice available - which likewise definitely implies that occasionally the rice will not be that ideal to eat all alone, so why egg seared was developed. It's a basic recipe with a great deal of space for modifying, with whatever meat and veg were left from the previous evening's dinner - so don't feel like you need to adhere to it inflexibly.

Ingredients:

- 2 eggs, beaten
- 1 cup white rice
- 1/2 cup frozen peas
- 3 carrots, cubed
- 2 tablespoons vegetable oil
- 4 tablespoons light soy sauce, 1 or 2 tbsp. as per taste

Method:

- Cook the rice as per bundle bearings and put it in a safe spot.
- Heat the carrots in water on medium-high heat for 5 minutes.
- Add the peas and mood killer the heat then drains the carrots and peas.

- Heat a wok or container over high fire, add the vegetable oil, carrots and peas and cook for 30 seconds before pouring the eggs.
- Mix to blend well.
- Blend in the rice and the light soy sauce and mix to cover the rice.

86: Smoked Haddock with Lentils and Spinach

A heavenly and simple recipe to cook Smoked Haddock with Lentils and Spinach. Its smoky flavor and firm surface work out positively for lentils, have an unrivaled flavor, and hold together when cooked, making them an ideal side dish. Don't be tricked by the straightforwardness of this dish, it packs in a lot of flavors making it a delectable and rapid midweek fish dish.

Ingredients:

- 1 stick celery, finely chopped
- 1 tsp olive oil
- 1 garlic clove, squashed
- 70g/2½oz tinned depleted brown or green lentils
- 100g/3½oz smoked haddock, boneless, skinless
- 40g/1½oz baby spinach
- 1 medium free-roaming egg
- 1 little onion (50g/1¾oz stripped weight), finely cleaved

Method:

- Heat the oil in a medium griddle and cook the onion and celery for 3–4 minutes.
- Add the garlic and lentils and cook for one more moment.
- Add 3 tablespoons of water and the spinach and cook for 5 minutes, adding more water if fundamental.
- In the interim, place the fish in a little griddle, cover it with water, and heat it to the point of boiling.
- Reduce the heat and stew for 5 minutes, or until the fish is cooked.
- Fill 33% of a little pot with cold water and heat to the point of boiling.
- Break the egg into a little bowl, then delicately tip it into the stewing water.
- Gently poach for 3–4 minutes.
- Reduce with an opened spoon and drain on kitchen paper.
- To serve, spoon the lentils onto a plate, then top with the fish and poached egg.

87 Pork with A Creamy Mushroom Sauce

Soup is the topmost loved with regards to starters and tidbits. It is both sound and hydrating as a result of its high water content. It can likewise remain as a feast without help from anyone else - simply set up a creamy soup, pair it with a cut of bread or two and you're all set.

Pork with A Creamy Mushroom Sauce benefits more than the taste buds. On account of its high water and fiber content, it helps flush with trip unsafe poisons from the body without being no picnic for the stomach. This is likewise the motivation behind why it's a successful dish to help one with shedding pounds - the water it contains helps one with topping off immediately contrasted with other food.

Ingredients:

- 1 teaspoon Seasoning salt (conform as you would prefer)
- 4 pork slashes, bone-in or boneless (around 1-inch thick)
- 1/3 teaspoon broke black pepper
- 2 tablespoons unsalted margarine
- 2 tablespoons olive oil
- Creamy Mushroom Sauce:
- 1 tablespoon fresh slashed thyme
- 1 cup cut brown mushrooms

- 4 cloves garlic squashed
- 2 tablespoons fresh cleaved parsley, separated
- 3/4 cup decreased fat cream or creamer, (weighty cream or vanished milk)

Method:

- Season cleaves with preparing salt and pepper.
- Heat oil and margarine in a griddle or pan over medium-high until the spread is dissolved.
- When the dish is hot, burn hacks for around 3-4 minutes for each side until brilliant seared and the middle is not, at this point radiant pink (fry in bunches if you need to).
- Move to a warm plate. Put in a safe spot.
- Add the mushrooms to the rich juices in the pan and cook for 3-4 minutes over medium heat.
- Scrap up any pieces extra from the hacks.
- When mushrooms are seared, add half parsley, half thyme, and the entirety of the squashed garlic; sauté for 30 seconds until fragrant.
- Pour in the cream and bring to a delicate stew for 3-4 minutes until marginally thickened.
- Season with salt and pepper, as you would prefer.
- Add the cleaves once again into the sauce, permit to stew briefly to warm through.
- Topping with outstanding spices and serve right away.

88: Lighter Spinach and Cherry Tomato Dal

This is a Lighter Spinach and Cherry Tomato Dal that my mother consistently makes. You can substitute various vegetables and greens and follow a comparable system. This is a generous and solid dish that leaves you fulfilled without packing you. You can substitute spinach for other dull greens like mustard greens, kale, or Swiss chard. The cook time will differ. Present with steamed rice.

Ingredients:

- ½ tsp curry powder
- 50g/1¾oz red lentils
- 1 tsp vegetable oil
- 20g/¾oz fresh ginger, stripped and finely cleaved
- 40g/1½oz child spinach
- 1 garlic clove, finely cleaved
- salt and freshly ground black pepper
- 8 cherry tomatoes, split
- 200ml/7fl oz. vegetable stock
- ½ little red bean stew, seeds reduced, finely slashed (or squeeze stew powder)
- 1 tbsp. slashed fresh coriander, to decorate
- 1 tiny red onion (50g/1¾oz stripped weight), finely chopped

Method:

- Heat the oil in a little pan over low heat.
- Add the onion, ginger, stew, and garlic, and cook for 3–4 minutes.
- Add the lentils, curry powder, and cherry tomatoes and cook for 1–2 minutes.
- Pour in the stock, bring to the bubble, then lessen the heat and stew for 15–20 minutes, or until the lentils are cooked, adding more stock if important.
- Stir in the spinach and season to taste.
- Boost with coriander and serve.

89: Cod in A Rich Tomato Sauce with Courgetti

Cod is only one of those popular fish species utilized in plans due to its white fragile living creature and sensitive flavor. Also, this fish is exceptionally nutritious; it is plentiful in vitamins (A, E, and D) and is a good source of omega 3 or that generally acclaimed unsaturated fat that is useful for the heart. Cod is low in cholesterol, which makes it useful for those with cardiovascular issues.

Ingredients:

- 1 plant tomato
- 1 tbsp. bean stew powder
- 1/2 Courgette slashed
- 1/2 red onion crushed
- 3 cloves garlic crushed
- 1/2 cup coriander crushed
- 3 tbsp. paprika
- 2 cod filets boneless and defrosted
- 2 tbsp. olive oil for broiling
- 2 jars chopped tomato or a jug of passata

Method:

- Wipe off the fish and season with a touch of salt, pepper, and a little paprika on the two sides.
- Leave it in the ice chest while you make your sauce.

- For your pureed tomatoes start by tenderly searing some crushed garlic, after about a brief add some crushed onions, half of the coriander, and the remainder of the paprika.
- Mix and let it fry tenderly.
- If you are utilizing chopped tomato, mix it heretofore.
- Pour in the passata and cleaved courgettes and season with the chilies, stockpot, pepper, blend well ensuring the stockpot is dissolving.
- Cover and let it stew
- When the courgettes are nearly cooked through, turn the heat to a low and delicately place your fish in the pan in a solitary layer.
- Cover with the chopped tomatoes set the top back on and let it cook for around 10 minutes until the fish is cooked.
- Trimming with the remainder of the coriander and serve hot with some stunning basmati rice or dried-up bread. It functions admirably with both.

90: Chicken with Ratatouille Bake

It's one of those adaptable plans that can go with any dinner. It fits totally on the smorgasbord table or richly masterminded on singular serving plates. It's consistently a success and you can change the ingredients to whatever you have available. It works for vegans and vegans. Furthermore, the extras can generally be utilized in different plans like plates of mixed greens or top a plain pizza outside for Mediterranean-style pizza.

Ingredients:

- ½ (1-lb.) eggplant, stripped and cleaved
- 1 little red onion, slashed
- 2 little summer squash, cleaved
- 2 tablespoons olive oil
- 2 garlic cloves, crushed
- 1 medium tomato, diced
- 1 medium-size red chime pepper, chopped
- ¼ cup chopped fresh basil
- ¾ teaspoon freshly ground pepper, separated
- 1 ¼ teaspoon legitimate salt, separated
- 6 (4-oz.) chicken breast cutlets
- 1 cup canola oil
- ⅓ cup generally useful flour
- Trimming: fresh basil leaves

Method:

- Sauté onion and eggplant in hot olive oil in a big nonstick pan over medium-high heat 5 minutes or until delicate and light brown around edges.
- Add squash, garlic, and chime pepper; sauté 5 minutes or until delicate.
- Add basil, tomato, and 1/4 tsp. every legitimate salt and freshly ground pepper.
- Cook, mixing continually, 2 to 3 minutes, or until the blend is completely warmed.
- Reduce vegetable combination from pan.
- Cover freely with aluminum foil to keep warm. Wipe pan clean.
- Wash chicken, and wipe off. Sprinkle with 1 tsp. salt and 1/2 tsp. pepper.
- Dig chicken in flour, shaking off overabundance.
- Fry chicken, in 2 groups, in hot canola oil in the pan over medium-high heat for 2 to 3 minutes on each side or until brilliant brown and done.
- Drain on a wire rack on paper towels. Cover & keep warm.
- Move to a serving dish, and top with the vegetable blend.

91: Low-Calorie Cottage Pie Recipe

Low-Calorie Cottage Pie with Chickpea Mash recipe is introduced underneath. Bungalow Pie and Shepherd's Pie are the same. Shepherd's Pie is produced using sheep through Cottage Pie utilizes hamburger. In this form of Cottage Pie, we utilize freshly crushed hamburger, anyway you can likewise utilize extra Roast Beef.

Ingredients:

- 1 onion
- 1 tablespoon of oil
- 1 carrot
- 500 grams of meat mince
- 1 tablespoon of pureed tomatoes (ketchup)
- 2 tablespoons of flour
- 1/2 to 1 tablespoon of Worcester sauce
- 1 bouquet garni or pack of spices slashed finely and one entire bay leaf
- ½ cup of peas
- 3/4 to 1 cup of meat stock
- 3 to 4 big potatoes
- 1 tablespoon of margarine
- salt and pepper
- ½ cup of corn parts (optional)

Method:

- Strip and slash the onion and carrot.
- Heat the oil in a big fry container or saucepan, add the onion and cook until the onion is clear.
- Add the crushed hamburger utilizing a wooden spoon to separate the mince.
- When the mince is completely sautéed mix through the flour and cooks briefly.
- Add the pureed tomatoes, carrot, peas, Worcester sauce, corn, and spices.
- Mix completely to join.
- Next, add the stock and bring it to the bubble.
- Reduce the heat and cover, stewing for 10 to 15 minutes.
- Add salt and pepper to taste.
- Strip the potatoes, hack, and spot in a sauce container with cold water simply covering the potatoes.
- Add somewhat salt to the water and bring to the bubble.
- Reduce the heat for 10 to 15 minutes or until the potatoes are delicate.
- Pound the potatoes with one tablespoon of margarine until the potato is creamy.
- Add salt to taste.
- Preheat the broiler to 190°C.
- Spoon the mince blend into a pie dish, then spoon or line the creamy squashed potato over the mince.

- Sprinkle ground cheddar on top whenever wanted and prepare for 15 to 20 minutes or until the potato is brilliant and the pie is warmed through.

92: Chicken and Cashew Noodle Stir-Fry

Sautéed food is an overall term that covers a particularly expansive scope of dishes. With insignificant planning time and only a couple of flavorings, one can create something extremely proficient and noteworthy. It is maybe one of the principal dinners that are educated in cookery classes, and especially mainstream among college understudies due to the low-planning time and sheer simplicity of making it. Today I'd prefer to acquaint you with the most loved Chicken and Cashew Noodle Stir-Fry recipe.

Ingredients:

- 1 tsp sugar
- 2 tsp corn flour
- 1 tbsp. oil
- 0.5 cup cashews, toasted
- 450 g Hokkien noodles
- 0.25 cup MAGGI Oyster Sauce 275mL
- 400 g chicken breast filet, cut
- 1 cloves garlic, squashed
- 0.25 cup water
- 100 g snow peas, top and followed
- 1 bundle child bok choy, cut

- 1 cup cut mushrooms
- 2 tsp MAGGI Original Seasoning 200mL

Method:

- Cook noodles as indicated by bearings on the package, drain.
- Join corn flour, Maggi premium shellfish sauce, Maggi unique flavoring, water, and sugar, put in a safe spot.
- Heat oil in a wok or big pan over high heat; add chicken, brown well.
- Add garlic, snow peas, and mushrooms, pan sear for 1 moment.
- Add sauce blend, noodles, bok choy, and cashews, pan sear until all-around consolidated and warmed through.

93: Quick Chicken Stew

Fast Chicken Stew recipe can help you with killing abuse and abundance spending with regards to giving solid, generous dinners for your family. With a little venture of time, you can begin redirecting cash from your basic food item spending straightforwardly into your blustery day reserve.

With a little piece of the creative mind, you can transform the Quick Chicken Stew recipe into healthy, delightful admission for your family. You can even manage your basic food item charge a part when you execute strategies that empower you to reduce family meat utilization. So, everybody feels better, and you have more cash in your wallet for sure.

Ingredients:

- 3 cloves garlic, crushed
- 1 stem celery, slashed
- Fit salt
- 1 tbsp. universally handy flour
- 2 tbsp. margarine
- 3 branches fresh thyme
- 1 cove leaf
- Freshly ground black pepper
- 3/4 lb. baby potatoes, quartered
- 3 c. low-sodium chicken stock
- 1/2 lb. boneless skinless chicken breasts
- Freshly slashed parsley, for decorating

- 2 big carrots, stripped and cut into coins

Method:

- In a big pot over medium heat, soften margarine.
- Add celery carrots, season with pepper and salt.
- Cook, blending regularly, until vegetables are delicate, around 5 minutes.
- Add garlic. Cook it around 30 seconds until fragrant.
- Add flour and mix until vegetables are covered, then add chicken, cove leaf, thyme, potatoes, and stock.
- Season with salt and pepper.
- Carry the combination to a stew and cook until the chicken is not, at this point pink and potatoes are delicate 15 minutes.
- Reduce from heat and move chicken to a medium bowl.
- Utilizing two forks, shred chicken into little pieces and get back to the pot.
- Boost with parsley before serving.

94: Sicilian Fish with Sweet Potato Chips

Cooking with fish shouldn't be overwhelming. If you understand what you'll cook at home, you'll have a thought of how the filets or the entire fish should wind up in a pot. However, if you are as yet figuring out how to cook, it is a good idea to stay with the most effortless plans for fish. This Sicilian Fish with Sweet Potato Chips recipe gives you fresh fish for just 177 calories and 8 grams of fat a serving. It's truly yummy with a sprinkle of malt vinegar.

Ingredients:

- 1 recipe Sweet Potato Chips
- ½ cup generally useful flour
- ¼ cup fat-free milk
- ¼ cup lager or nonalcoholic brew
- ½ teaspoon salt
- 1 egg
- ¼ teaspoon ground black pepper
- Malt vinegar
- ½ cup canola oil
- 1 pound fresh or frozen cod or halibut filets, around 1/2 inch thick
- Fresh parsley branches (optional)

Method:

- Plan Sweet Potato Chips. Defrost fish, whenever frozen. Put in a safe spot.
- For the player, in a medium bowl whisk together flour, milk, beer, egg, 1/2 teaspoon salt, and 1/4 teaspoon pepper until joined.
- Cover and chill hitter for 30 minutes.
- Lessen stove temperature to 250°F.
- Flush fish; wipe off with paper towels.
- Cut fish transversely into eight pieces.
- In an 8-inch pan heat canola oil over medium-high heat for 2 minutes.
- Plunge four bits of the fish in the player, going to cover and allowing abundance hitter to dribble off.
- Fry fish pieces in the hot oil for 4 to 6 minutes or until brilliant brown and fish chips effectively when tried with a fork, turning once part of the way through broiling time.
- Move singed fish to paper towels; let remain to deplete.
- Spot fish on a heating sheet; keep warm in the 250°F broiler.
- Rehash with the excess fish pieces.
- Serve fish with Sweet Potato Chips and malt vinegar.
- Whenever needed, decorate with parsley twigs.

95: Hoisin Salmon with Broccoli and Noodles

Make the most of your number one take-out-style dinner comfortable with this simple and better form of Hoisin Salmon with Broccoli and Noodles. Salmon and broccoli pan-seared in a profound brilliant without soy sauce and sprinkled with sesame seeds, served over a bed of cushioned white rice.

Ingredients:

- 1 lb. salmon cleaned, * cut into scaled-down pieces
- 1 Tbsp. canola oil
- 2 garlic cloves, crushed
- 2 Tbsp. low-sodium soy sauce
- 2 Tbsp. black or white sesame seeds
- 1/2 cup hoisin sauce
- 10 oz. uncooked rice noodles
- 1 little bundle of broccoli, cut into reduced down pieces (around 1/2 cup)

Method:

- Plan noodles as per bundle guidelines.
- Put in a safe spot.
- Steam broccoli until dazzling green and almost fork-delicate, around 4 minutes.
- Put in a safe spot.
- Heat oil in a nonstick pan (on a medium heat).

- Tenderly add salmon pieces.
- Cook salmon, undisturbed, until undersides of pieces, are brown, around 3 minutes.
- Flip salmon pieces.
- Add soy sauce, garlic, and broccoli to the pan.
- Cook until salmon pieces are cooked through, around 3 additional minutes.
- Delicately throw salmon and broccoli blend with cooked noodles.
- Sprinkle with hoisin sauce, decorate with sesame seeds and serve.

96: Prawn and Tomato Pasta

The pasta presented with a fine white wine makes a heavenly dinner. If red wine is your favorite drink, it is as great as that as well. Pasta is a particularly adaptable staple; I use it at least a few times each week. I have a major family, and pasta is awesome nourishment for when you're on a careful budget.

Contingent upon what you serve the pasta with, it tends to be a significant dinner in itself. If presenting with fish or prawns, it is sufficient pasta for six to eight-person. If serving all alone, it serves four to six-person without any problem.

Ingredients:

- 3 cloves garlic
- 250g fettuccine
- 1/2 white onion, cut into wedges
- 4 tablespoons olive oil

- 3 tablespoons fresh oregano leaves
- 4 medium tomatoes, slashed
- 1 squeeze salt and pepper to taste
- 3 tablespoons cleaved fresh basil
- 1 cup spinach leaves
- 250g fresh mozzarella, diced
- 500g cooked prawns - stripped and deveined

Method:

- Heat a big pot of delicately salted water to the point of boiling.
- Add the pasta and cook for 8 minutes, or until delicate. Drain.
- In the compartment of a food processor consolidate the garlic, onion, and oregano.
- Heartbeat until finely cleaved.
- Heat the olive oil in a big frypan over medium heat.
- Add the onion combination; cook and mix until fragrant and practically brilliant.
- Blend in the tomatoes, basil, salt, and pepper.
- Stew for around 5 minutes while the pasta is cooking, blending at times.
- Blend in spinach until it withers, then not long before the pasta is done stir in the prawns.
- Cook until warmed through.
- Throw with pasta in a big serving bowl and blend in mozzarella cheddar.

97: Jerk Pork with Sweet Potato Mash

This recipe sneaks up all of a sudden with flavor as well as will give you a portion of supplements as a result. Pork is perhaps the best source of thiamine, vitamin B1. Thiamine is essential by the way we make energy in our cells.

It is required as a cofactor in the initial step of high-impact breath and needed to make synapses like acetylcholine and reuse one of the significant cancer prevention agents in our bodies, glutathione.

Yams, additionally give us a good source of magnesium, potassium, and beta carotene. I'm likewise offering my simple Jerk Pork to Sweet Potato Mash recipe below.

Ingredients:

- 1½ tsp runny nectar
- 2 tsp jerk preparing
- 1 tsp olive oil
- 300g/10½oz pork tenderloin
- 100ml/3½fl oz. pineapple juice (from 227g tin pineapple rings)
- 1 x 350g/12oz yam, stripped and cut into 3cm/1¼in pieces

For the Salsa:

- 2 tbsp. generally cleaved fresh coriander leaf
- 3 spring onions, daintily cut

- ½ lime, squeeze as it were
- ½ red bean stew, deseeded and finely diced
- 1 tsp olive oil
- squeeze salt
- 2 tinned pineapple rings (about 100g/3½oz), depleted and finely cleaved

Method:

- Blend the jerk preparing, nectar, and pineapple juice in a shallow bowl adequately big to hold the pork.
- Add the pork flank and spot in the ice chest, covered, for at any rate 30 minutes or overnight, turning the pork a few times.
- Preheat the stove to 200C/180C Fan/Gas 6 and line a heating plate with kitchen foil.
- Reduce the meat from the marinade, saving the fluid, and pat it dries with kitchen paper.
- Warmth the oil on a high heat.
- Brown the meat on one side, turn over and brown on the opposite side.
- Spot the meat on the heating plate, pour over the marinade, and dish for 20–25 minutes, turning the pork over the following 15 minutes.
- Cut into the thickest piece of the steak to watch that it is delicious yet cooked through.
- Then, bring a pan of daintily salted water to the bubble and stew the yam for 15 minutes until delicate.
- Drain, squash, and season with salt and pepper.

- To make the salsa, blend the pineapple, coriander, spring onion, a press of lime juice, stew, olive oil, and salt in a bowl and put in a safe spot for in any event 10 minutes.
- Turn the meat over in its decreased marinade and leave to rest for 5 minutes.
- Cut the pork into 2cm/¾in-thick cuts and present with the squash and salsa.

98: Spanish Style Chicken Traybake

Traybakes make midweek dinners a breeze! This Spanish Style Chicken Traybake consolidates fresh chicken, chorizo, cook peppers, fresh potatoes, garlic, and paprika for most extreme scrumptious Spanish heavenliness with at least fight – only 15 minutes' involved time, and the broiler deals with the rest!

Ingredients:

- 2 red onions, each cut into 8 wedges
- 2 tbsp. olive oil
- 1/2 tsp. sweet smoked paprika
- 8 chicken thigh fillets
- 1 every red and yellow pepper, deseeded and cut
- 4 tomatoes, quartered
- 500 g child fresh potatoes, divided assuming big
- 125 g chorizo ring, cut into adjusts
- 50 g pitted black olives
- 1 tsp. dried oregano
- 2 garlic cloves, squashed
- 50 ml fino or manzanilla sherry, optional

Method:

- Preheat stove to 200°C imprints 6. Throw the onions, oil, potatoes, and some flavoring in a big cooking tin.

- Cook for 30min.
- Cut the highest point of every chicken multiple times and sprinkle over the paprika and a lot of freshly ground black pepper.
- Blend the peppers, tomatoes, chorizo, olives, and garlic into the cooking tin and sprinkle over the oregano.
- Set the chicken on top and add the sherry, if utilizing.
- Keep cooking for 40-45min, seasoning the chicken halfway through with any juices in the pan.
- Present with a fresh green plate of mixed greens and some bread to clean up the juices, if you like.

99: Zesty Chili Steak Fajitas

Fajita is for the most part hamburger, chicken, pork, or shrimp barbecued and served on a flour tortilla with sauces. Fajita is served to the table sizzling boisterously on a metal platter with tortilla and sauces as an afterthought.

Ingredients:

- 4x flour tortillas
- 1x red ringer pepper
- 1x medium-big onion
- 1x yellow ringer pepper
- 1x tablespoon of Cajun zest
- 12oz of good quality rear-end or sirloin steak

Method:

- Residue the crude steak(s) in the Cajun powder and a little sprinkle of olive oil.

- Get your hands filthy for the best outcomes.
- Permit the steaks to sit for around 5 minutes and afterward place on a hot BBQ (make sure the flares have faded away).
- Cook the steaks for around 5-10 minutes relying upon how well you as them done.
- Add the peppers and onion, turning them for two or three minutes.
- Make sure everything is singe flame-broiled and lookin' scrumptious.
- Reduce from the BBQ onto a slashing board and cut everything into slight strips.
- Do the steak last since we need to keep in the heat.
- Fill your steak fajitas to the edge, adding a fresh green plate of mixed greens or guacamole and acrid cream or salsa.
- I love to add a teaspoon of tabasco into my salsa for that extra *kick*.
- Make the most of your steak fajitas with a fiery red wine, a cool ale, or fresh lemonade.

100: Simple Veggie Chili

This Easy Veggie Chili is a basic recipe that doesn't need a lot of planning and difficult work. The time I spend on tasks or school work possesses expanded significantly while the energy for me to investigate fresh plans is scant.

Consequently, it is essential to cook something speedy and simple to plan. This recipe unquestionably fulfills the models for "fast and simple". You can appreciate a quality dinner in only 15 minutes with no problem.

Ingredients:

- 1 (8 ounces) Tomato Sauce
- 2 (14.5 ounces) Diced Tomatoes Chili Ready with Onions
- 1 (10 ounces) frozen entire bit corn
- 1 (15 ounces) black beans, washed and depleted
- 2 teaspoons stew powder
- 1 (15 ounces) garbanzo beans, washed and depleted

Method:

- In a big pot, join tomatoes, garbanzo beans, pureed tomatoes, black beans, corn, and stew powder; blend well.
- Heat to the point of boiling over medium-high heat.
- Decrease heat; cover and stew for around 10 minutes.
- Spoon bean stew into singular soup bowls.

101 Pork Stir Fry Recipe

Here's a good method to utilize pork tenderloin to make a Mexican-style feast in a brief timeframe. Here's a tip: You can defrost the corn rapidly by placing it in a colander and running warm water over the corn.

Ingredients:

- 3/4 pound of pork haunch
- olive or vegetable oil
- 1/2 cup thick salsa
- 1 medium onion - cut into flimsy wedges,
- 2 garlic cloves – crushed
- 1 little red ringer pepper - cut into strips
- 2 cups frozen corn - defrosted,
- 1 little zucchini - cleaved
- 1 can black beans - depleted and washed

Method:

- In a big pan, heat 1 tablespoon of oil over medium-high heat until hot.
- Include the pork strips, ringer pepper, onion, and crushed garlic.
- Cook and mix for 6 to 8 minutes or until the pork are not, at this point pink.
- Stir in the corn, black beans, slashed zucchini, and salsa.

- Cover and cook on stew for 5 minutes, or until the zucchini is fresh and delicate.
- Sprinkle with salt and pepper as wanted.

102: Chorizo Beans On Toast

This Chorizo Beans On Toast recipe is an astonishing dinner. It's profoundly prepared meat that implants each nibble of these beans with stunning flavor. It was the ideal method to raise these beans to the following level and make them extra scrumptious. Toast some great bread, sprinkle with olive oil, and rub with a clove of garlic. Then, top the toast with the prepared beans, alongside some fresh cilantro, a crush of lime juice, and, if you need, some disintegrated queso fresco or cotija cheddar.

Ingredients:

- 1 fresh narrows leaf
- 2 chorizos, thickly cut
- 2 tbsp. extra-virgin olive oil, in addition to extra for showering
- 200 gm canned cherry tomatoes
- 1 little Spanish onion, meagerly cut
- 800 gm canned white beans, depleted, flushed
- 180 ml (¾ cup) chicken stock
- 1 tbsp. Sherry vinegar, or to taste
- 8 thick cuts sourdough bread

- 2 oregano branches, in addition to adding leaves to serve
- 1 garlic clove, finely chopped, in addition to 1 additional clove, split, for scouring

Method:

- Heat oil in a pot over medium-high heat, add chorizo, and mix every so often until cooked (1-2 minutes).
- Add onion and garlic and mix every so often until delicate (3-4 minutes), stock and spices, add beans, tomato, season to taste, and stew until fluid is very much enhanced and reduced considerably (4-5 minutes).
- Reduce spices, add vinegar, and season to taste.
- Then, preheat barbecue to high.
- Sprinkle bread cuts with a little oil and barbecue, turning once, until brilliant (1-2 minutes each side).
- Rub with cut-side of garlic, top with bean combination, dissipate with oregano and serve hot

103: Con Carne with Guacamole

These are the most famous varieties of Chilies. However, the stew isn't just a zesty and delicious feast. It is useful for your wellbeing, as well. The Chili Peppers utilized in the plans are plentiful in vitamin C and it appears they have numerous ideal impacts on wellbeing. Its zest upholds absorption, gives a characteristic hunger, and fortifies the wellbeing of the internal organs.

Ingredients:

- 1/4 cup in addition to 3 tablespoons corn oil
- 1 pound dried pinto beans, doused by bundle bearings
- 3 1/2 pound plum tomatoes (around 18)
- 10 garlic cloves (skins left on)
- 2 1/2-pound medium yellow onions (around 7), stem closes managed, quartered the long way with skins left on
- 3 ancho chilies
- 4 Mulato chilies
- 1 can (14 1/2 ounces) low-sodium meat stock
- 5 pounds ground round or ground throw
- 1 cup water
- 1 tablespoon coarse salt
- 1/2 teaspoon freshly ground black pepper
- 2-ounce Mexican chocolate or semisweet chocolate slashed
- Knotty Guacamole

Method:

- Drain and wash the doused beans, and spot in a big pan with water to cover by 2 inches.
- Heat to the point of boiling, lessen heat, cover, and stew delicately until beans are delicate around 1/2 hours.
- Heat 2 tablespoons oil in a 12-inch cast-iron pan over medium heat; add tomatoes, and cook, turning at times, until skins start to scorch, around 5 minutes.
- Cover pan, reduce heat to medium-low, and keep on cooking, turning, until tomatoes have relaxed, 7 to 8 minutes more. Move to a big bowl.
- When adequately cool to deal with, strip and center tomatoes.
- Spot tomato substance in a perfect bowl, and hold.
- While tomatoes cool, place 66% of onion quarters in the same pan with 2 tablespoons oil.
- Cover, and cook over medium heat, turning sporadically, until pleasantly burned and mollified, 12 to 15 minutes.
- Move to a bowl to cool.
- Rehash with garlic cloves, remaining onion, and another tablespoon of oil.
- When sufficiently cool to deal with, strip garlic and onion, cutting off and disposing of roots and strips, and adding substance to the bowl with the tomato.
- Move vegetables and any juices to a blender in bunches and puree until almost smooth. Put to the side in a big bowl.

- Tear the chilies fifty-fifty, and dispose of stems and seeds.
- In a similar pan over medium heat, toast chilies in leftover 2 tablespoons oil, turning with utensils, until smoky, around 3 minutes.
- Move to the blender.
- Heat stock and water to the point of boiling, pour over chilies, and let remain until chilies are malleable around 5 minutes.
- Puree chilies and stock, and stir into tomato combination.
- In a 7-quart Dutch stove over medium heat, cook 33% of meat, separating it with a spoon and mixing incidentally until pleasantly sautéed around 8 minutes.
- While meat is cooking, brown another third of the meat in the pan.
- Then add that group to the first in the Dutch broiler.
- Mix tomato blend into meat in Dutch broiler.
- Brown leftover hamburger in the same pan; add to Dutch stove.
- Drain cooked beans.
- Add cooked beans to pot with salt.
- Heat the stew to the point of boiling, lessen the heat, cover, and stew delicately, blending, until heat is delicate and sauce is thick around 1/2 hours.
- Stir in chocolate, and season with pepper.
- Present with guacamole.

104: Chicken Satay Wraps

Chicken wings are the most un-expensive type of white meat accessible and are normally sodden and delicious. Sauces or marinades like the grill, prepared, hoisin, nectar mustard, teriyaki, or satay can acquaint wings with a universe of flavors. Residue wing areas with flour or corn starch then cover with your preferred sauce. Organize on an oiled heating plate and cook for 30 minutes in a 375-degree broiler.

Ingredients:

For the Satay:

- 2 cloves garlic, stripped and cut
- 1/2 tsp curry powder
- 12 eight-inch bamboo sticks (absorb water for 30 minutes before cooking)
- 1/2 tsp entire or ground coriander seeds
- 3 - 4 boneless skinless thighs or 2 boneless skinless chicken breasts
- 1/2 tsp turmeric
- 2 TB cleaved shallots
- 1 TB ginger, cleaved
- 1/2 cup coconut milk
- 3-inch piece of lemongrass, thick and extreme external layers reduced, cut daintily, and afterward crushed (optional; discard if the ingredient is hard to track down)

For the Sauce:

- 1/4 cup cleaved shallot
- 1/4 cup coconut milk
- 1 TB coconut oil
- 3 cloves garlic, cleaved
- 1 TB fish sauce
- 2 tsp lime juice
- 1/2-inch ginger stripped and cleaved
- 2 tsp red curry glue
- 1/4 cup any nut margarine or finely ground nuts... cashew, almond, walnut, and so forth... any nut or blend of nuts (aside from peanuts)

For the Cucumber Salad:

- 2 TB lime juice
- 2 TB cleaved fresh cilantro
- lettuce leaves (we utilized Bibb)
- 1/4 tsp salt or to taste
- 1 cucumber, stripped and cut into little dice

105: Vegan Chili

This tasty Vegan Chili recipe makes six empanadas. Regardless of whether you are cooking for vegans, everybody will adore this recipe for vegetarian empanadas. They are prepared instead of pan-fried. These make a filling starter recipe or a heavenly lunch or vegetarian nibble.

Ingredients:

- 1 medium red onion, slashed
- 2 tablespoons extra-virgin olive oil
- 1 big red ringer pepper, cleaved
- 2 ribs celery, cleaved
- 2 medium carrots, cleaved
- ½ teaspoon salt, partitioned
- 2 tablespoons stew powder
- 4 cloves garlic, squeezed or crushed
- 2 teaspoons ground cumin
- 1 teaspoon dried oregano
- 1 ½ teaspoon smoked paprika
- 1 big can (28 ounces) or 2 little jars (15 ounces each) diced tomatoes, with their juices
- 1 can (15 ounces) pinto beans, washed and depleted
- 2 jars (15 ounces each) black beans, washed and depleted
- 2 cups vegetable stock or water
- 1 bay leaf

- 1 to 2 teaspoons red wine vinegar, sherry vinegar OR lime juice (to taste)''''
- 2 tablespoons slashed fresh cilantro, in addition to extra for embellishing
- Tips: chopped cilantro, cut avocado, tortilla chips, sharp cream or crème fraiche, ground cheddar, and so forth

Method:

- In a big Dutch stove or substantial lined pot over medium heat, warm the olive oil until shining.
- Add the slashed onion, chime pepper, carrot, celery, and ¼ teaspoon of the salt.
- Mix to join and cook, mixing incidentally, until the vegetables are delicate and the onion is clear around 7 to 10 minutes.
- Add the garlic, bean stew powder, cumin, smoked paprika, and oregano.
- Cook until fragrant while blending continually, around 1 moment.
- Add the diced tomatoes and their juices, the depleted black beans and pinto beans, vegetable stock, and cove leaf.
- Mix to consolidate and allow the blend to go to a stew.
- Keep cooking, blending every so often, and lessening heat as important to keep a delicate stew, for 30 minutes.
- Reduce the bean stew from the heat and dispose of the sound leaf.
- For the best surface and flavor, move 1 ½ cups of the bean stew to a blender, making a point to get a portion of the fluid bit.
- Safely attach the cover and mix until smooth (keep an eye out for hot steam), then empty the mixed blend once again into the pot.

- Add the cleaved cilantro, mix to consolidate, and afterward blend in the vinegar, to taste.
- Add salt to taste, as well—I added ¼ teaspoon more now.
- Divide the combination into singular dishes and present with enhancements of your decision.
- This stew will save well in the cooler for around 4 days or you can freeze it for longer-term storage.

106: Breakfast Oatmeal Cupcakes

These adjustable breakfast heated cereal cupcakes are incredible in a hurry fuel for those occasions when you have zero time in the first part of the day to set up a major feast. You can undoubtedly switch around the flavor by picking various flavors and add-ins for perpetual breakfast cupcake varieties.

This recipe makes preparing with stevia fun and simple. You can make these sound prepared cereal breakfast cups early and stash them in the cooler for a fast and filling breakfast.

Ingredients:

- 5 cups moved oats
- 1 tsp salt
- 2 1/2 cups over-ready crushed banana
- 5 tbsp unadulterated maple syrup, agave, or honey OR stevia comparable sum
- 2 1/3 cups water - Increase to 2/3 cups if utilizing stevia
- 2/3 cup smaller than usual chocolate chips, optional
- 1/4 cup + 1 tbsp coconut or veg oil (45g)
- Optional add-ins: cinnamon, chopped pecans, smashed coconut, ground flax or raw grain, raisins or other dried fruit, and so forth
- 2 1/2 tsp unadulterated vanilla concentrate

Method:

- Preheat stove to 380 F, and line 24-25 cupcake tins.

- In a large blending bowl, consolidate every dry ingredient and mix well overall.

- In a different bowl, consolidate and mix every single wet ingredient (counting banana).

- Blend wet into dry, then fill the cupcake liners and heat 21 minutes. I also prefer to then sear for 1-2 minutes, however, it's optional.

- These cereal cakes can be consumed right, or they can be frozen and warmed for a moment breakfast on a bustling day.

Here is another incredible, without a wheat recipe. If you experience difficulty getting your children to have a sound breakfast, try this one. Expectation you and your family will appreciate these biscuits similarly as. These oats biscuits are produced using essential ingredients; such as ingredients you would have found in your grandma's washroom. However, being stacked with the supported energy of moved oats I have a little stunt that keeps them light and fleecy.

Ingredients:

- 1 cup whole wheat flour
- 1/3 cup sugar
- 2 teaspoons preparing powder
- 3/4 cup milk
- 1 egg
- 1/4 cup oil
- spread (genuine margarine) for the container
- 1/2 to 1 cup raisins
- 1 cup oats (moved breakfast oats), conventional sluggish (large) type

Method:

- Pre-heat a stove to 375°F.
- Spread a biscuit container or cupcake skillet.
- Spot the dry ingredients in a single bowl, and the wet ingredients in an alternate bowl.

- Blend the two dishes separated, then combine them and blend once more.
- Spoon hitter into the skillet.
- Cook for 20 minutes, or until brown with firm edges.
- Promptly turn the biscuits over utilizing a margarine blade. Leave them in the hot dish to keep the buildup from demolishing the surface.

Chia Seeds are a good source of fiber calcium, omega-3s, and iron. They likewise have limited quantities of phosphorous, manganese, potassium, and copper. I love their "crunchy" surface. They nearly help me to remember custard yet they're a lot better for you. Chia seeds can be eaten crudely or cooked.

I suggest eating them after they've either been drenched (like in a pudding recipe) or cooked because these seeds extend whenever they've been hydrated. Eating them dry can prompt them to extend in your throat which may give you a marginally abnormal inclination. One of the big advantages is the fiber content which will help give you a sensation of completion prompting better satiety.

Ingredients:

- 1/4 tsp vanilla embodiment
- 1 tsp. maple syrup
- 1 cup almond milk
- 1/4 cup white chia seeds (can use black)
- 1/2 cup characteristic Greek yogurt
- 1/4 tsp cinnamon
- 1/4 cup frozen OOB Organic blended berries

Method:

Into a little bowl, add chia seeds, yogurt, almond milk, honey, and vanilla concentrate

Mix well, as you don't need the chia to be staying together.

Cover, and leave in the ice chest short-term (or for 3+ hours).

Following two hours, give it another mix to guarantee it's all blending through.

Into a blender, add the chia combination (It should be thick at this point!) and the frozen berries.

Mix for 2-3 minutes, until your ideal consistency.

109: Eggplant Bacon

As a vegetable, eggplant doesn't have the best standing. However, this isn't because of the actual eggplant, this is a direct result of how it is habitually arranged. Breaded and singed, then layered with oily cheddar, eggplant unexpectedly turns into a caloric bad dream. The eggplant itself isn't high in calories, in any case.

It is comprised of 92% water and in this way contains just around 14 calories for every half cup all alone. It is likewise a good source of fiber, calcium, and potassium. So eggplant is an incredible decision to remember for your supper plate, and there are numerous sound and tasty approaches to set it up.

Eggplant sweethearts cheer—here's one all the more method to make the most of your number one purple-cleaned vegetable. Give this eggplant a shot crostino with a sprinkle of sliced tomatoes, feta, and tricks, or mix it into your #1 pasta with a sprinkle of good extra-virgin olive oil and a modest bunch of sliced basil.

Ingredients:

- Freshly ground black pepper
- 2 tbsp. extra-virgin olive oil
- 1 medium eggplant
- 2 tbsp. soy sauce
- 1/2 tsp. smoked paprika
- 1 tsp. maple syrup
- 1/2 tsp. Fluid Smoke

Method:

- Preheat broiler to 300°. Line 2 preparing sheets with material paper.
- Cut eggplant in quarters, longwise.
- Cut each quarter into long, flimsy strips.

- In a small bowl, whisk together soy sauce, olive oil, paprika, maple syrup, and fluid smoke.
- Spot eggplant cuts onto heating sheets and brushes the two sides with sauce. Season with pepper.
- Prepare until eggplant is cooked through and starting to get fresh, 45-50 minutes

110: Homemade Curry

Would you like to realize how to make simple curry that is loaded with healthy flavor and goodness that is modest and credible? Is it accurate to say that you are tired of paying great cash for exhausting and dull curries from your local cafés? Allow me to tell you the best way to make perhaps the best curry. All that curry can be an exquisite feast. A curry is ideal for supper or lunch. I have eaten numerous curries in my daily existence.

Unfortunately, I have eaten a lot of awful curries that have been made by individuals who should know better! A good curry shouldn't be costly. A good curry comprises fresh plans, spices, and flavors. The best thing about everything is that you will eat a homemade curry that is not difficult to make and is loaded up with sound spices and flavors.

Ingredients:

- curry leaf (10 leaves)
- ginger 2cm
- 300 grams of your #1 meat (marinate with a teaspoon of curry powder, sugar, teaspoon salt, and pepper for 2 hours before cooking)
- curry powder 300 grams

- 1 cup of coconut milk
- 1 teaspoon of pepper
- 50 grams dried chilies
- olive oil
- 2 garlic cloves
- 2 onions
- Indian Nan bread or supper bread rolls

Method:

- Heat a frying skillet with olive oil. Whenever it's warmed then add the garlic, curry leaf, onions, and ginger and mix until brilliant.
- Add your meat and mix for 2 minutes.
- In a 20-liter pot, add every one of the ingredients and cook for 2 hours under low heat.
- Mix the pot like clockwork to help the ingredients blend and keep the lower part of the pot from consuming.
- Add the coconut milk toward the end and carry it to the bubble.
- To thicken the curry if it's not too much trouble, add cornflour in a little bowl and add a large part of some water.
- Blend this and afterward empty it into the pot and mix until the curry thickens.
- Topping with some fresh cream and coriander.

111: Bean Stew Seasoning

Potentially the least demanding because the essential ingredient is for some odd reason bean stew powder. Some you aware of everything might be thinking "Hello, bean stew powder is one of those pre-fabricated blends of a few flavors!" and you would be right however bean stew powder is fundamentally flavors and practically zero filler.

So back to the recipe, the stew powder will give you the bean stew flavor, then to add some profundity and smoky flavor we will add ground cumin, then you can add got dried out onions, garlic powder, and some other ingredient you think would round out the flavor profile that you need to make. There are a lot of plans for making "stew" preparing on the web.

Ingredients:

- 1 teaspoon cocoa powder
- 3 tablespoons bean stew powder
- 1 tablespoon ground cumin
- 1/2 teaspoon garlic powder
- 1/2 teaspoon onion powder
- 1/4 teaspoon cayenne pepper
- 1/2 teaspoon red pepper drops
- 1/4 teaspoon ground cinnamon
- 1 teaspoon paprika (use smoked paprika for a smokey contort)

Method:

- Combine all ingredients as one in a little bowl or container. Store in a little sealed shut holder.
- In the wake of cooking meat and vegetables for bean stew, mix in flavor blend and toast for 1-2 minutes before adding fluid ingredients to stew.

The incredible thing about utilizing dates in your cooking is that it is flexible. You can use it in its strong state, as a thick puree, or in fluid-structure! You can use pretty much, contingent upon your preferences. Before utilizing dates in cooking plans consistently make sure that you pit them.

That implies eliminating the seed from within. It is not difficult to do and because the fruit is dry on the surface, there is no wreck included. Since the external skin of a date will in general solidify, particularly in cool environments, one valuable tip is to splash for a couple of moments in barely enough warm water. This isn't compulsory for all plans.

Date syrup is a well know sugar accessible today. Old cuneiform original copies from Mesopotamia notice the syrup, showing it as the essential sugar of that time. Thinking about the significant amount of date palms around there, it is likely this was alluding to honey from the date, or, date syrup.

Ingredient:

- 20 Medjool dates pitted
- 3 cups water

Method:

- Put the dates and water in a medium pot on medium-high heat to heat to the point of boiling.
- Then turn the heat down to medications low and let the blend stew.
- If you see froth showing up on the top, skim it off (the same thing you do when making soup broth, or jam).

- Utilizing a wooden spoon, blend sporadically and crush the dates with the rear of the spoon.
- After around 15 minutes of stewing, take it off the heat and let it cool.

113: Sirloin Steak

Sirloin steaks can give large cuts from 1.5 inches (37mm) to 2 inches (51mm) thick and are found to be for the most part the least expensive of the superior steaks. This is the reason this steak is generally well known among men and genuine grills. It is supposed that the name 'sirloin' was subsequently an English lord who was enamored with quality food and knight a piece of meat which he names 'sir midsection'. However, this is likely a miss-truth!

It is a unique sort of steak produced using hamburger meat that has been scaled from the back or back bit of the cow into its short flank. It includes the most sensitive and delectable meat a piece of the said creature, making it truly outstanding among the various steaks like t-bone, porterhouse, club steak, and such.

Ingredients:

- black pepper
- vegetable oil, or groundnut oil
- 2 sirloin steaks, estimating 3cm in thickness
- 1 handle of spread
- 1/4 pack of thyme
- flaky sea salt
- 3 garlic cloves, slammed yet unpeeled

Method:

- Before you start, reduce the steaks from the ice chest and let to come to room temperature (for at any rate 60 minutes)
- Preheat the stove to 180°C/gas mark 4
- Spot a substantially based skillet or iron dish over high heat and add a good scramble of oil.
- Season the steaks generously with flaky ocean salt
- When the oil is hot, add the steaks cautiously to the skillet and cook for 2 and a half minutes, or until wonderfully brilliant on the underside.
- Turn the steaks over and add a handle of spread, some thyme, and a couple of garlic cloves. Cookie the steak with the margarine and once brilliant on the underside, place on the stove for 2–3 minutes
- Reduce the steaks from the skillet and let to rest in a warm spot for 5 minutes before serving. Season and serve

114: Cereal Banana Waffle

A waffle is a kind of cake like a hotcake. They are for the most part prepared between two hot plates. Cooking the two sides simultaneously. This gives them an inside and out crunchy outside and a uniform tone. They are the most broadly had breakfast food on the planet. The fan top pick anyway is the Oatmeal Banana Waffle. It very well might be a direct result of its abundant resources that trap products of the soil so you get a ton in one chomp.

Ingredients:

- 2 cups water
- 2 cups oats
- 1/2 banana
- 2 tablespoons olive oil
- 2 tablespoons powdered milk
- 1/2 teaspoon salt

Method:

- Turn waffle iron on high
- Put ingredients in the blender and mix on high until the substance are smooth
- Allow the blend to sit for a couple of moments to thicken
- Shower the waffle iron with a non-poisonous non-stick splash
- Pour the blend on to the waffle iron
- Cook for around 10 minutes
- Rehash until you are out of the player

115: North Staffordshire Oatcakes

North Staffordshire oatcakes are a local delicacy in the North Staffordshire space of England, thus might be referred to non-local people as a North Staffordshire oatcake or Potteries oatcake. These utilize flour and yeast, though different oatcakes don't.

When pre-cooked, they are a type of inexpensive food, and catering outlets in the space generally offer oatcakes with fillings like cheddar, bacon, wiener, and egg. They can be re-warmed by fricasseeing in margarine, or by flame broiling.

What's more, pikelets are frequently served close by oatcakes also.

Ingredients:

- 8oz fine oats
- 1 teaspoon salt
- 8oz whole-wheat or plain flour
- 1/2oz fresh yeast
- 1 teaspoon sugar
- 1/2 pints' warm milk and water, blended cream

Method:

- Add the salt to the flour and oats.
- Break up the yeast with somewhat warm fluid and add the sugar. Let the blend get foamy.
- Blend the dry ingredients with the yeast fluid to make a hitter.
- Cover the hitter with a spotless material and leave it in a warm spot for 60 minutes.
- Prepare the oatcake on an all-around lubed iron. Put sufficient player onto the frying pan to create an oatcake around 8-9 creeps in breadth. The surface will be canvassed in openings as it cooks.
- Turn the oatcake following 2 - 3 minutes when the upper side seems dry and the under is brilliant brown, and cook for another 2 - 3 minutes.

116: Cereal Raisin Cookies

The word 'oats raisin cookies' carries water to the mouth and fills the nostrils with its warm smell. Allow us to examine the recipe of oats raisin cookies, how grandmother used to make, with a slight variation. Since many keep away from eggs but then many are sensitive to drain items, we will get ready vegetarian cereal raisin cookies.

The flavor challenges depiction and the fragrance of them heating will transform even the most current of kitchen spaces into a Donna Reed-time cooking retail outlet. Don't be amazed if you end up battling the staggering desire to tie on a gingham cover while the blending and preparing measure happens.

Ingredients:

- 1/3 c water or milk
- 1/2 tsp vanilla
- 1/4 c brown sugar - immovably stuffed
- 3/4 c spread, fruit purée, a balance of margarine and vegetable oil, or shortening
- 1 egg
- 3c oats, moved (crude) - fast/antiquated
- 1/2 tsp heating pop
- 1 c flour - universally handy
- 1/2 tsp salt
- 1c raisins
- 3/4 c pecans - sliced
- 1/4 tsp cinnamon

Method:

- Heat broiler to 350°F.
- Delicately oil cookie sheet with oil.
- Consolidate margarine, fruit purée, spread/vegetable oil blend, or shortening, brown sugar, milk, egg, and vanilla; beat with the blender on fast to mix well.
- Consolidate oats, flour, heating pop, salt, and cinnamon; add to the shortening combination and join until just mixed.
- Mix in raisins and nuts.

- Drop by adjusted tablespoonful onto lubed cookie sheet, 2 inches separated.
- Prepare for 10-13 min., or until gently cooked.

There is certainly something exceptional about a Chai Tea Latte. For individuals who are stuck in a rut and who need to adhere to moment espresso or normal tea that might be a genuine disgrace because without taking a stab at something fresh, you don't have the foggiest idea of what you are absent. It is in every case great to try fresh things throughout everyday life.

It is extraordinary being somewhat gutsy with your food and beverages, although I would resist the urge to stress about the hard beverages. Chai tea latte is a quieting drink arranged without any preparation using a chai combination. Furthermore, we have arranged a few stages to make a reviving beverage of chai tea latte.

Ingredients:

- 2 black tea sacks (optional; I like to use Darjeeling)
- 2 cups almond milk (or milk of decision)
- 3/4 teaspoon ground cinnamon, or to taste
- 1/4 teaspoon ground ginger
- 3 tablespoons maple syrup (or sugar of decision)
- 1/8 teaspoon ground cloves

Method:

- In the case of utilizing tea, remember that this beverage will have caffeine.
- Heat the almond milk in a pot over medium-high heat, until it starts to rise around the edges of the skillet.

- Mood killer the heat, and add the 2 tea packs to the pot of hot milk.
- Hang tight 3 to 5 minutes for the tea to steep, then reduce the packs and proceed with the following stage.
- In case you're skirting the tea, add the plain almond milk to a sauce skillet.
- Since the milk is in the pot (regardless of whether it's been blended as tea, or not) include the cinnamon, cloves, ginger, and maple syrup.
- Race to join, mixing over medium heat, until the blend is steaming hot.
- Change any flavoring as you would prefer and serve right away.
- Extras can be store in a water/airproof compartment for as long as 4 days in the refrigerator.
- You can serve them chilled over ice, or warm on the oven once more.

Everyone likes granola bars yet did you realize that they are really basic and modest to make at home? When you make homemade granola bars you can tweak the flavor and surface to suit your specific preferences and you can make them as nutritious or wanton as you can imagine.

The recipe is essential and just requires a couple of moments of hands-on readiness followed by a speedy outing through the stove. Toward the end, you have a tremendous plate of heavenly tidbits that will save pleasantly in a covered holder for at any rate seven days. By exploring different avenues regarding ingredients you can make fresh flavors and surfaces.

Ingredients:

- 3 eggs
- 1/3 cup brown sugar (discard if granola is extremely sweet)
- 3/4 cup softened spread or margarine
- 1 teaspoon vanilla
- 1/2 teaspoon salt
- 4 cups granola cereal

Method:

- Preheat the broiler to 400 degrees. In a blending bowl, combine as one softened margarine and sugar.
- Add vanilla, salt, and eggs.
- Beat until smooth.

- Mix in granola and press into a lubed 9x13 heating dish.
- Heat in the broiler for 15 to 20 minutes or until all-around set.
- Cool and cut into bars.
- These are flat-out genuine cookies and particularly pleasant if you have made a strawberry or peach jam throughout the mid-year.
- In this after recipe, carob powder is used.
- Carob is regularly called 'the chocolate substitute." It makes prepared products dull and damp.
- It is produced using the case of the carob tree, also called St. John's bread.

119: Chocolate Brownie

Such a Chocolatey chocolate brownie that must be accomplished by good natural cocoa and chocolate. Such a Chocolatey chocolate brownie that increases in flavor if you leave them in a tin for a little while. This recipe also bends over as a hot pudding for a cold winter's day, it is brilliant hot with frozen yogurt over it, however, use an espresso or vanilla frozen yogurt as a rich chocolate one takes away from the kind of the brownie.

Ingredients:

- 250g spread
- 300g caster sugar
- 3 large natural eggs in addition to an extra egg yolk
- 250g chocolate

- 60g flour
- ½ tsp preparing powder
- 60g great quality natural cocoa powder

Method:

- Oil the preparing plate with margarine.
- Put the sugar and spread it into the bowl of a food blender and cream them together for a few minutes until they are pale and feathery.
- Put a bowl over a dish of boiling water, yet make sure that the lower part of the bowl doesn't contact the water, or the chocolate will go grainy when it dissolves.
- Keep 50g to the side and break the rest into little parts and leave it in the bowl over the water.
- Leave it for five minutes and mix, when it has liquefied reduce it from the heat.
- Break the excess 50g into pieces the size of big full raisins.
- Beat the eggs gently in a little bowl.
- Strainer together the flour, cocoa, and heating powder to reduce the irregularities and make it light and vaporous, add a spot of rock salt to escalate the kind of chocolate.
- Add the eggs to the creamed spread and sugar a little at a time, it will sour if you add everything simultaneously.
- When the egg has all been fusing, overlap in the liquefied chocolate and the chopped chocolate.

- Delicately overlap in the flour and cocoa, do this gradually, and don't exhaust, as you should be certain not to take the air out of the flour blend.
- Fill the readied dish or heating tin and shake on the worktop, to level the top marginally.
- Heat for around thirty minutes, the chocolate brownies are prepared when the edge is pulling somewhat away from the dish, however, the middle looks delicate and squiggly.
- If you don't know embed a metal stick in the middle and it should arise marginally wet, however not with crude combination adhering to it.
- Brownies proceed to cook and set in the tin when cooling so make sure that it isn't overcooked.
- If it isn't exactly prepared, return it to the stove yet check each a few minutes.

120: Taco Seasoning

Tacos are scrumptious and are made to go with lunch and supper, or similarly as a side dish if you like to. Then you can add tomato, onion, sharp cream, fresh guacamole and you can finish off it with anything you like. Imagine how delectable these tacos will be and they will be caused with all the stuff you to feel are astounding together.

Ingredients:

- 5 teaspoons paprika
- 6 teaspoons bean stew powder
- 4 1/2 teaspoons cumin
- 3 teaspoons onion powder

- 2 1/2 teaspoons garlic powder
- 1/4 teaspoon cayenne pepper

Method:

- Join all ingredients together, and blend well. This should be store in a water/airproof compartment for as long as a half year.
- You can change this recipe, here and there I like to add some oregano to my blend.
- Smoked chipotle peppers and ancho pepper are likewise pleasant increments, as they will make heavenly flavors.
- Perhaps the best thing about making your zest mix is that you will change and alter the recipe for your preferences.
- If you like zesty food, you can add more cayenne pepper. If you don't care for it so fiery, you can avoid the cayenne pepper about the recipe.
- To use this flavoring blend, basically use 3 tablespoons and some water whenever you have sautéed one pound of ground hamburger.
- Essentially add the flavoring blend, and water, and let the water decrease by 1/2 and you have a few tacos that have been prepared impeccably, and you did it all yourself without purchasing a business blend.

121: Mama yo (Vegan Mayonnaise)

Delightful vegetarian mayo, made with just 4 ingredients and in only 2 minutes! This vegetarian mayonnaise is so scrumptious, velvety, rich, and without cholesterol. Making vegetarian mayo is so natural, it just requires 4 ingredients, only 2 minutes, and a blender, there's nothing more to it.

A submersion blender is the most ideal decision; however, a normal blender will do. This vegetarian mayonnaise is made without milk or eggs. It tastes incredible as a plunge with veggies or on bread. Store in a shut compartment in the cooler for as long as about fourteen days.

Ingredients:

- 1/2 tsp salt
- 1/2 cup unsweetened soy milk (125 ml)
- 1 cup oil (250 ml)
- 2 tsp apple juice vinegar

Method:

- Make sure the oil is at a similar temperature as the milk. You can use cold oil and cold milk, however, I discovered room temperature milk and oil to be the simplest to work with.
- In case you're utilizing an inundation blender, join every one of the ingredients in the blender cup, place the submersion blender in, so way it sits solidly on the lower part of the cup, and heartbeat until the mayo emulsifies.
- When the greater part of the veggie lover mayo has emulsified, you can move the blender here and there to consolidate any oil that is perched on the top.

- In case you're utilizing a standard blender, place every one of the ingredients in the blender, except the oil, and mix for around 5 seconds.
- Then add the oil progressively while the blender is going at a sluggish speed until it thickens, then you can divert it steadily from low to high and let it go until all around blended.
- Try the mayo and add more salt if necessary. If it's excessively thick, add more milk, and if it's too watery add more oil.
- Heartbeat again until the mayo has the ideal consistency.
- Use it promptly or save it in the refrigerator for a couple of hours until it's cold. Keep extras in a water/airproof compartment or a container in the refrigerator for around 4-7 days.

122: Taco Stuffed Peppers

This speedy and simple supper recipe makes certain to satisfy the whole family! Peppers loaded up with the best taco meat, finished off with cheddar, and the very best taco ingredients. In case you're longing for tacos however not all the carbs, you'll love these eased-up stuffed peppers.

The peppers are burrowed out and simmered in the stove, then loaded down with ground hamburger, black beans, brown rice, corn, and salsa. It's beginning and end you love about tacos, all in a consumable vegetable bowl. You can generally trade ground meat for chicken or turkey, or stick to rice and keep this recipe vegan.

Ingredients:

- extra-virgin olive oil
- 1 clove garlic, crushed
- 1/2 Onion, sliced (around 1 cup)
- 1 lb. ground hamburger
- Freshly ground black pepper
- adequate salt
- 2 tbsp. Sliced cilantro
- 1/2 tsp. ground cumin
- 1 tsp. bean stew powder
- 1/2 tsp. smoked paprika
- 1 c. smashed Cheddar
- 3 ringer peppers, split (seeds reduced)
- 1 c. Smashed Monterey Jack
- Hot sauce, for serving
- 1 c. Smashed lettuce
- Pico de gallo, for serving
- Lime wedges, for serving

Method:

- Preheat the broiler to 375° and splash a big heating dish with a cooking shower.
- In a big skillet over medium heat, heat around 1 tablespoon olive oil.
- Add onion and cook until the onion is delicate around 5 minutes.
- Mix in garlic. Cook it until fragrant

- Add ground meat and cook until not, at this point pink, around 5 minutes. Channel fat.
- Add ground cumin, bean stew powder, and paprika to hamburger blend, then season with salt and pepper.
- Sprinkle ringer peppers with olive oil and season with salt and pepper.
- Spot the peppers, cut side up, in the heating dish, and spoon meat combination into each pepper.
- Top with cheddar and prepare until the cheddar is liquefied and the peppers are fresh delicate, around 20 minutes.
- Top each pepper with lettuce and present with pico de gallo, hot sauce, and lime wedges.

123: Chicken Tagine with Prunes and Almonds

Food in Morocco assumes a significant part in customary life. From weddings to sanctifications to circumcisions, it is the premise of get-togethers and festivities. From couscous to tagines and pastilles, the fragile flavors are a mix of tastes of numerous human advancements. A conventional Moroccan dish is a tagine, a stew of vegetables with poultry or meat and dried fruit.

The fruit is added towards the finish to give general pleasantness to the dish. The vegetables are set around the meat, which is set in the focal point of the pot along with the fruit. The tagine is then covered and cooked gradually over a charcoal oven

Ingredient:

- 1 chicken, cut up into 6 pieces

- 170 g (6 oz) dried prunes, chopped fine
- 60 g (2 oz) whole, whitened almonds
- 1 large white onion, finely sliced 2 cloves of garlic, squashed
- ½ teaspoon powdered ginger
- 1 teaspoon powdered cinnamon
- ½ teaspoon turmeric
- 1 teaspoon ground cumin
- 2 tablespoons vegetable oil
- salt and freshly ground black pepper to taste

Method:

- The following, set up the chicken marinade.
- Wash the chicken in salted water and channel.
- Blend squashed garlic in with 1 tbsp. salt to make glue.
- Rub into the chicken and afterward flush under running water until the chicken no longer scents of garlic.
- Channel and store.
- Rub the chicken pieces with cumin, salt, and pepper and let represent 60 minutes.
- Cover the prunes with cold water, add the cinnamon and bring to the bubble.
- Cover and stew for 30 minutes or more - until the prunes are delicate.
- Spot the chicken pieces in a 5-quart profound meal over medium heat and add the chopped onion, ginger, turmeric, salt, pepper, and almonds.
- When the almonds are brown, reduce with a punctured spoon and

- channel on kitchen paper.
- When the chicken is seared, cover with water just so the chicken pieces are covered and bring to the bubble.
- Reduce heat and stew, covered, for 30 minutes.
- Following 30 minutes, add the prunes and a part of the prune water to the goulash and keep cooking until the chicken and prunes are extremely delicate.
- Sprinkle with the almonds and serve on the double.

124: Lemon Iced Tea

Tea has no calories, however, it has heaps of cancer prevention agents in fundamental basic Fresh tea, and even it will assist you with losing weight. To get the nutritious employments of it you need to try it at home as per your taste. Here is a healthy summer seasoned tea plan and enhanced frosted tea syrups and you can likewise make unsweetened tea recipes.

Making tea is peaceful and simple; you can drink it light or healthy, drink it without sugar or with sugar. Whenever you have the basics, you can begin getting innovative - simply follow the simple strides beneath. You can use seasoned frosted tea sacks.

Ingredients:

- 1 ¼ cups sugar
- 2 big lemons
- 2 cups fresh mint leaves, in addition to additional for decorating
- ½ cup fresh lemon juice
- 6 black tea packs

Method:

- Utilizing a vegetable peeler, reduce dazzling yellow strip from lemons.
- Join lemon strip and sugar in a medium pan with 1/2 cup water and heat to the point of boiling, blending to break up sugar.
- Lower heat and stew for 2 minutes.
- Reduce from heat and mix in mint.
- Cool to room temperature; strain.
- Steep the tea packs in 4 cups of bubbling water, covered, for 5 minutes.
- Then reduce tea packs.
- Mix in syrup, 4 cups cold water, lemon squeeze, and ice healthy shapes.
- Serve in tall glasses loaded up with ice and a couple of mint leaves.

125: Ratatouille

Comprised of a wide range of vegetables, ratatouille is generally tantamount to a vegetable stew. An adaptable dish by its own doing: it tends to be served hot, cold, or even tepid. Consider it an hors d'oeuvre, consider it your principal course, anything you desire to call it, it's an exemplary French dish, to be specific from the Provencal district.

Some serve it with fundamentals, others on a bed of rice. Ratatouille bears no weight of limitations. Furthermore, for all you extra darlings, many fight that ratatouille tastes better the day after it is cooked. Chocolate and Zucchini even consider it an "ideal make-ahead dish." So give it a shot.

Ingredients:

- 1/4 cup olive oil, in addition, to add on a case by case basis
- 1 little eggplant, sliced
- Legitimate salt and freshly ground black pepper
- 1 zucchini, chopped
- 3 little tomatoes, chopped
- 1 pepper (red, green, or yellow), sliced
- 1 onion, sliced
- 3 cloves garlic, squeezed
- 3 or 4 leaves fresh basil, sliced
- 2 teaspoons sliced fresh thyme
- Sprinkle red wine vinegar

Method:

- Heat 2 tablespoons of oil in a large skillet or Dutch broiler.
- Cook the vegetables each in turn (independently) for 5 to 7 minutes, adding somewhat more oil on a case by

case basis and preparing with salt, in the accompanying request: onion, zucchini, eggplant, pepper, and tomatoes.

- Consolidate the whole of the cooked vegetables together in the skillet, thyme, add the garlic, and basil and let stew delicately for 20 minutes.
- Add a sprinkle of red wine vinegar, season with salt and pepper, and afterward turn off the heat.
- Serve hot, warm, or cold.

126: Avocado Egg Cups

Although avocados start from Mexico and Central America they were purchased to Spain by the conquistadors and have adjusted well to the Mediterranean environment and develop here in bounty. They are a surprising and valuable fruit since they don't as expect mature until picked so can be left on the tree and be gathered throughout the whole year.

Already they have been found to have umpteen medical advantages and as they are incorporated routinely in the Mediterranean diet they give further weight to the well-being giving advantages of this diet.

Ingredients:

- 6 big whole egg
- 3 Avocado
- 6 cut Uncured Turkey Bacon

Method:

- Slice the main avocado down the middle and scoop out the seed. Scoop out a part of the avocado to make space for the eggs.
- Rehash these means for the excess two avocados.
- Preheat the broiler to 425 degrees Fahrenheit.
- Spot the avocado parts on a biscuit tin and break 1 egg in every avocado.
- Heat for 14 to 16 minutes, or until the eggs are cooked as you would prefer.
- Top with cooked, uncured turkey bacon - one strip for every avocado half.

127: Scaled Down Frittatas

There is by all accounts a touch of conversation about what a frittata (articulated 'free-TAH-tah) truly is. Is it a kind of quiche, or is it an omelet? To give the initial two definitions, a quiche regularly is an egg dish made with cream prepared in an outside layer, practically like a pie. A quiche can have an assortment of ingredients added into it to make various styles and tastes.

An omelet, on the other hand, is just beaten eggs cooked with spread or oil in a griddle with the hardened egg collapsed around different ingredients. Average omelet ingredients incorporate cheddar, onions, bacon, mushrooms, different vegetables, ham, or different meats.

Frittatas can contain quite a few unique ingredients. Fresh vegetables, mushrooms, cheeses, meat, potatoes, various spices, or any mix thereof are normal. Extra vegetables or cooked meat are likewise incredible in frittatas. Spices, fresh or dried, can likewise add a great deal of flavor to a frittata, or you could use your number one hot pepper sauce to zest it up too.

Ingredients:

- 3/4 cup salsa
- 1-1/2 cups frozen smashed hash brown potatoes, defrosted
- 1 Italian turkey hotdog connect (around 4 ounces), packaging reduced
- 1/2 cup chopped onion
- 1 teaspoon canola oil
- 1/3 cup water
- 1 garlic clove, crushed
- 1/2 teaspoon salt
- 1/2 to 1 teaspoon dried oregano
- 1/4 teaspoon pepper
- 3 large eggs
- 1/2 teaspoon dried thyme
- 2 big egg whites
- 2 tablespoons universally handy flour
- 1 cup buttermilk
- 1/4 cup smashed Parmesan cheddar

Method:

- In a nonstick skillet, cook frankfurter over medium heat until not, at this point pink.
- Reduce with an opened spoon to paper towels. Dispose of drippings.

- In a similar skillet, sauté potatoes, onion, and garlic in oil until potatoes are brilliant brown, around 5 minutes.
- Add water, flavors and hotdog; cook and mix over medium heat until the water has vanished, around 1 moment.
- In a bowl, consolidate the eggs, egg whites, buttermilk, flour, and Parmesan cheddar.
- Mix in hotdog combination. Fill biscuit cups covered with cooking splash three-fourths full.
- Prepare at 350° for 20-25 minutes or until a blade confesses all.
- Thoroughly run a blade around the edge of cups to extricate frittatas.
- Present with salsa.

128: Pasta and Summer Vegetables Recipe

If you read my recipe for Tomato Salad, you realize that I love the late spring. I trust you do likewise. Throughout the late spring, everything is simply blasting around you. Vegetables are at their pinnacle of readiness and flavor. Everything is simply so acceptable. You never consider wintertime and the lower evaluation of vegetables that are accessible. If you have a nursery, you can develop all that is in this dish. Hence, it will be greatly improved.

Ingredients:

- 1 Medium Zucchini
- 3 Large, Blood Red Native Tomatoes
- 1 Medium Onion. Red, Yellow or White
- 1 Yellow Squash
- Garlic Cloves
- 7 Fresh Basil Leafs, Torn
- Olive oil, salt, and pepper
- Hard Italian bread
- ½ pounds of dry pasta
- Ground Parmesan cheddar

Method:

- Carry a Large Pot of water to the bubble. Salt the water generously and cook the pasta until Al Dente. Somewhat hard.

- While trusting that the word will bubble and keeping in mind that the pasta is cooking, do stages 2-9
- Coarsely Chop the Tomato, store
- Slice the zucchini down the middle the long way and afterward into equal parts longwise once more. Coarsely cleave, store
- Do likewise for the Yellow Squash, store
- Coarsely dice the onion, store
- Coarsely slash the garlic, store
- In a griddle on medium/high, sauté the onion and garlic until marginally delicate.
- Spot the Zucchini and Yellow Squash in with the onion and garlic. Sauté until marginally relaxed
- Yet, the tomatoes in the griddle and sauté until mollified marginally
- Spot the pasta in the griddle alongside 1-2 Ladle's of pasta water
- Cook everything on Medium/High heat until the vegetables are marginally more relaxed. 3-5 minutes
- Mood killer them and toss in the basil and throw.

129: Green Beans and Almonds

Fresh green beans should be fresh and break effectively when they are bowed. If the green bean creases over effectively it isn't just about as fresh as it should be. It can in any case be used however the freshness of the bean is no more. There isn't anything more delectable than great fresh green bean plans and I will give you a part of my top picks.

Before I get into the plans I might want to reveal to you how you can freeze fresh green beans. Spot the beans in a sifter and whiten with extremely boiling water. Quickly place the beans in a plastic cooler pack and spot them in your cooler on the rack where you would put all moment freeze food sources.

Ingredients:

- 1/2 stick of spread
- 2 lbs. of fresh green beans
- 1 cup of toasted almonds less if you don't care for a lot of almonds
- Salt and pepper to taste

Method:

- Wash and reduce the string from the green beans and snap off the finishes.
- Bubble or steam the green beans until cooked yet fresh
- In a skillet dissolve the margarine and add the cooked green beans
- Blend well and add the almonds and salt and pepper.
- Combine the whole of the ingredients as one well and on a low fire let the combination
- Cook until done however the beans are as yet fresh.

130: Chicken Pork Adobo

Being perhaps the most loved food variety of Filipinos, the adobo has a few varieties. The chicken pork adobo is a recipe that is consistently present in the weekly menus of families since it is a mix of two of the most cherished meats for the Pinoy sense of taste.

It also works to the upside of mothers who get befuddled between pork adobo and chicken adobo because there is no more need to settle on a decision between the two. For my situation, my better half loves pork adobo while my child consistently demands chicken adobo. To fulfill them both, I generally wind up cooking chicken pork adobo as well.

Ingredients:

- 3 tablespoons salt
- 1/4 pounds' pork flank broil (boneless and cut into 2-inch pieces)
- 1/4 pounds' chicken bosoms (boneless, skinless, and cut into 2-inch pieces)
- 2 cloves garlic (crushed)
- 2 inlet leaves (torn)
- 2 tablespoons squashed garlic
- 1 tablespoon black peppercorns (coarsely ground)
- 1 tablespoon vegetable oil
- 1 cup white vinegar
- 1/4 cup soy sauce (optional)

Method:

- Use salt and pepper to prepare the chicken and pork meat.
- Then put all the meat in a broth pot. Add the torn cove leaf and squashed garlic.
- Coat with white vinegar and soy sauce.
- Cover the pot and spot it in the cooler for at any rate 8 hours or overnight to marinate.

- Cook under medium-high heat and heat to the point of boiling.
- Then decrease heat and stew until meat is delicate when tried with a fork, as a rule, takes around 1 ½ hour.
- To prevent drying out, add a little measure of water whenever required.
- Reduce the meat from the cooking fluid.
- Spot the fluid back to the broth pot and let stew.
- Over medium-high heat, cook the meat in vegetable oil while mixing.
- Continue cooking until every one of the sides of the meat becomes brown.
- Just now after cooking, add the leftover crushed garlic.
- Add every one of the meats to the stewing fluid and cook until the sauce is marginally thickened.
- Serve hot with plain white rice.

131: Best Veggie Broth

Vegetable broth is an economical and healthy approach to add flavor to a wide range of suppers. Save extra vegetables, scraps, and spices in a big cooler sack until you have enough to make the stock. Examination with various vegetable mixes to track down the best flavor. Freeze broth in more modest segments for simple and fast access. Broth can be frozen in an ice 3D shape plate and afterward moved to cooler packs.

Ingredients:

- 8 cups water
- 1 inlet leaf
- 2 medium onions, cut into wedges

- 2 tablespoons olive oil
- 2 celery ribs, cut into 1-inch pieces
- 3 medium leeks, white and light green parts just, cleaned and cut into 1-inch pieces
- 1 whole garlic bulb, isolated into cloves, and stripped
- 1/2 pound fresh mushrooms, quartered
- 1 cup pressed fresh parsley branches
- 1 teaspoon salt
- 3 medium carrots, cut into 1-inch pieces
- 4 branches fresh thyme
- 1/2 teaspoon whole peppercorns

Method:

- Heat oil in a stockpot over medium heat until hot.
- Add celery, onions, and garlic.
- Cook and mix for 5 minutes or until delicate.
- Add leeks and carrots; cook and mix for 5 minutes.
- Add water, parsley, mushrooms, salt, peppercorns thyme, and cove leaf; heat to the point of boiling.
- Lessen heat; stew, revealed, 60 minutes.
- Reduce from heat.
- Strain through a cheesecloth-lined colander; dispose of vegetables.
- In the case of utilizing quickly, skim fat. Or on the other hand, refrigerate for 8 hours or overnight; reduce fat from the surface.
- Broth can be concealed and refrigerated for 3 days or frozen as long as a half year.

132: Creole

Tomatoes and shrimp concocted with garlic and onions - this Gulf Coast custom will make them long for the narrows. This recipe can either be a fundamental dish or a side dish. You can make it as hot as you need, simply add more stew powder and hot sauce. Serve over hot rice. This Creole dish is cooked with tomatoes, onions, peppers, and celery. Change the zest to your inclination, yet don't be frightened of a little heat.

To the plan of the best jambalaya recipe, here is a customary Creole Jambalaya recipe that will undoubtedly stimulate the taste buds.

Ingredients:

- About 142grams of chicken cut them into about 2.5cmsq. 3D shapes
- 2 and ½ cups of rice
- About 85grams of pork ribs, cut the same size as the chicken. Smoked pork doesn't work!
- About 170grams of Andouille hotdog suggested yet replacements will do if inaccessible in the nearby market
- About 142grams of ham healthy shapes
- About 343grams of crude shelled shrimps
- 1 and ½ cups of finely sliced onions
- A 0.35l of hand squashed tomatoes, an unquestionable requirement!
- 1/2 cup of finely sliced red chime pepper
- 1 cup of finely sliced celery

- 1 cup of finely sliced green chime pepper
- 6 cloves of squashed or squeezed garlic
- Clam or vegetable juice, depending on the situation - No water!
- 2 cups of chicken broth
- ½ tablespoon every one of white, red, and black peppers
- ¼ teaspoon of finger-squashed saffron
- 1 tablespoon of pale dry sherry, whenever wanted
- ¼ teaspoon of monosodium glutamate
- ¼ teaspoon of thyme
- 3 tablespoon of Spanish olive oil, an absolute necessity
- 1 and ½ teaspoons of Hungarian HOT paprika
- 1 little cove leave

Method:

- Heat the olive oil in the Cast Iron Pot or a Dutch stove
- Add the peppers, onion, garlic, and celery and mix, cook on high flares until ingredients are clear
- Add the chicken and pork and continue to mix until they become white
- Add the Ham and wiener and mix for about 3minutes
- Add the tomatoes and mix for 5minutes
- Lower the heat to medium and add the chicken broth and mix
- With the same heat, add a wide range of various flavors aside from the sherry in any request and mix.
- Let to cook for about 20minutes.
- Add the rice

- Cover the pot
- Cook for about 30minutes
- Add the shrimp and the sherry
- If necessary or if the rice isn't all around cooked, add the Vegetable or Clam squeeze and mix it all. Let to cook for another 5 to 10minutes
- Mood killer the heat and let it stew and serve

133: The Ultimate Acai Berry

The ubiquity of the Acai Berry Smoothie is obvious; indeed, you can see it advanced anyplace, from chocolates, juices, lunchrooms, and even wellbeing drinks. You would now be able to make your own Acai smoothie. It very well may be effortlessly arranged and it is ideal for your wellbeing.

If you are experiencing difficulty getting your children, or even yourself, to eat or drink whatever's healthy for them, why not let them try this. You can get every one of the advantages of the berry from this beverage and it is the ideal method to get going your day and give you that additional charge you need.

The ingredients are not definite, yet just estimated since you need to think about your taste when making this. Aside from that, as long as you put in the berries, then you can choose the amount of what you will add. This recipe serves around two individuals, so you can make so a lot or as little as you need.

Ingredients:

- Void two Acai cases into it or a teaspoon of acai powder.

- 6-7 strawberries
- 1/2 cup blueberries
- 2 scoops of non-fat vanilla frozen yogurt

Method:

- Put the strawberries and the blueberries in the blender.
- Mix them until they are smooth, except if you need to have some chunkier pieces.
- Add the two scoops of vanilla frozen yogurt into the blender, and mix away alongside the berries.
- Open two containers of the Acai and empty the substance into the blender under a low setting.
- This will help with guaranteeing an intensive blend.
- And afterward, the whole of that is left is a major good glass of Acai smoothie only for you.

134: Marinara Sauce Recipe

Here is an extraordinary recipe for marinara sauce utilizing canned tomatoes. This marinara sauce is delectable over your #1 pasta, on top of pizza, and over mussels and shrimp. The excellence of this sauce is that it tends to be used with various plans, so it's an extraordinary beginning stage in Italian Cooking and it is not difficult to make.

You can use either fresh or canned plum tomatoes for this recipe, anyway utilizing fresh tomatoes requires additional time and planning, so I like to use canned. If you do anticipate utilizing fresh tomatoes, make certain the tomatoes are ready and in season.

For the canned tomatoes, I lean toward Rienzi brand tomatoes. I have tried various brands of canned tomatoes and Rienzi has the best flavor among the grocery store brands, as I would see it.

Ingredients:

- 1/4 cup extra virgin olive oil
- 1 35-ounce jar of whole plum tomatoes with fluid
- 4 garlic cloves, stripped and sliced (More or less relying upon the amount you like garlic)
- Salt to taste
- 10 - 12 fresh basil leaves, torn
- Squashed red pepper to taste
- 1/2 teaspoon of dried oregano

Method:

- Open your container of tomatoes and squash them by hand into a bowl and store.
- Medium heat the olive oil in a big pan.
- Add your garlic to the oil and cook until delicate and daintily sautéed.
- Make sure to watch the garlic to ignite sure it doesn't.
- Cautiously add the tomatoes alongside their fluid into the dish with garlic and oil.
- Use alarm while adding the tomatoes to the hot oil. The oil can splatter.
- Add the oregano.
- Mix the blend and heat to the point of boiling.
- Season with a touch of salt and red or black pepper.

- Lower the heat so the sauce is reduced to a stew.
- Separate the tomatoes as it cooks with a spoon until your sauce is thick.
- You need the sauce to stew until thickened, around 20 - 25 minutes.
- Add your fresh basil a couple of moments before the sauce is finished.
- Taste the sauce
- Add more salt or pepper if necessary.
- Serve over your favorite pasta.

135: Pesto Sauce Recipe

This is another extremely simple and delightful recipe that can be served over your number one pasta, grilled chicken, mussels, or as an ingredient for pizza. For a good minor departure from this recipe, have a go at adding sundried tomatoes to the pesto combination before mixing for a delectable tomato pesto sauce.

This recipe is a guide for you. Not every person has similar inclinations. Some don't care for a lot of garlic or olive oil flavor for instance, so it is suggested that you try until you track down the correct recipe.

Ingredients:

- 3/4 cup sliced pecans or pine nuts (the nuts can be daintily toasted in a dry skillet before mixing for added flavor)
- 4 cups fresh basil leaves
- 2 cloves garlic, stripped and chopped (pretty much relying upon your taste)
- 1/2 cup of extra virgin olive oil
- 1/2 cup of ground Parmesan cheddar
- salt and pepper to taste

Method:

- Add all ingredients to blender (except olive oil.)
- Add a little oil at once until sauce arrives at the wanted consistency.

Prepared to serve in your number one dish.

136: Simple Pasta with Garlic, Oil, and Fresh Herbs

This is another fast and simple Italian recipe with a couple of ingredients. Significantly, you don't consume the garlic with this recipe else it will turn out to be harsh.

Ingredients:

- 1 pound of spaghetti
- 1/2 cup held pasta water
- 3 - 4 garlic cloves sliced
- 1/4 Cup of Chopped Italian Flat Leaf Parsley
- 6 tablespoons of extra virgin olive oil

- 1/4 cup of sliced fresh basil leaves
- A spot of red pepper pieces
- Salt to taste

Method:

- In a large pot, achieve 6 quarts of salted water to a moving bubble.
- Add the pasta and cook for around 6 - 8 minutes or until still somewhat firm.
- Channel however make sure you save around 1/2 cup of pasta water.
- Heat 4 tablespoons of olive oil (while the pasta is cooking) over medium heat in a large skillet.
- Add the garlic and sauté until light brown in shading.
- Make sure to give close consideration to the garlic to ignite sure it doesn't.
- Reduce from heat.
- Mix in fresh spices, red pepper drops, and few tablespoons of the saved pasta water.
- Blend until joined.
- Move the depleted pasta to a big serving bowl and blend in the excess olive oil and pasta water.
- Add the garlic and spice combination into the pasta and blend well.
- Taste and add salt and red pepper whenever wanted.
- Serve right away. Top with ground cheddar whenever wanted.

137: Sicilian Succo

Ground hamburger and ground pork meatballs are seared in olive oil and served over a rich pureed tomato in this conventional Sicilian recipe. You can substitute zucchini for the meatballs for a veggie lover variant.

Ingredients:

- 1 tsp garlic powder
- 3 (29-oz) jars pureed tomatoes
- 4 cloves garlic (chopped)
- 4 (6-oz) jars tomato glue
- 1 tbsp chopped fresh basil (fresh)
- 1 tbsp chopped parsley (fresh) + extra 1 tbsp
- 2 lbs ground meat
- 1 cup dry bread pieces
- 1 lb ground pork
- 1 cup ground Parmesan cheddar

Method:

- In a big pot, blend the sliced garlic, pureed tomatoes and glue, 1 tbsp parsley, and basil.
- Heat this sauce to the point of boiling, then turn the heat down to low to stew the sauce.
- In a bowl, combine as one the pork, hamburger, bread morsels, parmesan cheddar, 1 tbsp parsley, and garlic powder.
- Combine this as one well, then structure into balls generally the size of a golf ball.

- Fry the meatballs in a skillet in hot olive oil until they are altogether cooked.
- Add the meatballs to the sauce blend and cover.
- Let it stew on low for around four hours.
- Serve over noodles of your decision.

138: Tiramisu

Perhaps the most mainstream cookies that can guarantee itself as an extraordinary top pick among everything is the Italian Tiramisu. Each café that serves Italian food makes certain to have it on its menu. Tiramisu was conceived distinctly in the 1970s in Veneto, Italy. It acquired prominence all through the world a lot later just in the mid-nineties.

This pastry contains ingredients that don't seem to mix well with one another however when used to the correct extents comes out as a lip-smacking sweet. Every one of the ingredients is so not quite the same as one another that, astonishingly, a particularly superb desert can be acquired when these ingredients are blended in the legitimate extents. Every one of these ingredients is sweet without help from anyone else.

Ingredients:

- 1/2 cup sweet Marsala wine
- 1 lb Mascarpone cheddar at room temperature
- 6 egg yolks
- 1/2 cups heated water
- 1/2 mug espresso seasoned alcohol
- 5 tsp moment espresso powder

- 12 ounces' ladyfingers or cut wipe cake
- Unsweetened cocoa (for cleaning)
- 1 cup sugar
- 1-ounce semi-sweet chocolate (ground) - optional

Method:

- In a bowl, blend 1/2 cups of heated water with the moment espresso.
- Mix until the espresso has broken up, then add the alcohol.
- Dunk in 1 ladyfinger at a time, quickly turning it to cover.
- Reduce it from the fluid and spot it on the lower part of an 8 x 8-inch dish. Line all espresso-covered ladyfingers one next to the other until a large part of the skillet's base is covered.
- Pour half of the mascarpone cheddar (or cream cheddar blend) over the highest point of the ladyfingers.
- Add another layer of covered woman fingers and cheddar.
- Refrigerate this for around 4 hours, or until the sweet is firm.
- Not long before serving, dust the top with cocoa.
- Embellish with the ground semi-sweet chocolate (whenever wanted) and slice into squares to serve.

Chapter: 11 Salad Dressing Recipes

139: Tomatoes and Sweet Onion Dressing

Tomatoes and sweet onion with Roquefort dressing is a conventional Italian salad that effectively loans itself well to

Italian dinners like Osso Bucco and lighter meals, for example, salad and Minestrone. Mainstream Italian eateries, for example, Olive Garden serve comparative dinners of soup and salad. The excellence of this Italian salad is that it is flexible to the point that it tends to be presented with pretty much any dinner.

Ingredients:

- Sweet onions
- Ready tomatoes
- Essential Italian Dressing
- Roquefort cheddar
- Green scallions
- Dried oregano
- Pepper
- Salt

Method:

- Cut ready red tomatoes and sweet onions exceptionally dainty.
- Spot four tomato cuts on each plate.
- Over the highest point of the tomatoes lay the onion cuts.
- Sprinkle super Basic Italian Dressing.
- Spot the two green scallions along the edge of the plate.
- Disintegrate the Roquefort cheddar over the top and sprinkle with dried oregano.
- Season to taste with salt and pepper.

Tahini sauce is an incredibly adaptable dressing that is an ideal supplement to everything from sandwiches to rice, pasta, and even meat dishes. Yet, perhaps the best blending is with fresh vegetables, which are changed from standard to exceptional with a delightful Lemon Tahini Dressing. This lemon tahini dressing is not difficult to make this delectable. It's creamy with a tart lemon flavor and goes so well with all your favorite salads.

Ingredients:

- Black pepper to taste
- 2/3 to 3/4 cups water (depending on the situation)
- 1/2 cup tahini
- 3 tablespoons fresh lemon juice
- 1 tablespoon olive oil
- 1 clove garlic, crushed
- 3/4 teaspoon ocean salt (or to taste)

Method:

- Whisk or mix all ingredients, beginning with 2/3 cup water and adding more until you arrive at an ideal consistency.
- The dressing will hold 5 to 6 days in the fridge.

141: Super Cabbage Juice

Do your children wrinkle their noses at the name of the vegetable? Well, that isn't generally excellent information as it is vital to remember cabbage for your child's diet. This tough and solid vegetable is bountiful in dietary benefit. It is plentiful in Vitamin A, B, C, and E and ensures your eyes and skin, improves your digestion, assists with consuming fat, and is a powerful enemy of oxidant. If your kids won't eat the vegetable, you can evaluate cabbage soup recipes of various types and have confidence your children will smack their lips.

Ingredients:

- 3 carrots
- 6 green onions
- 2 green peppers
- 1 container of mushroom
- 2 jars of tomato
- A lot of celery
- 1 package of Lipton soup blend
- Half top of a cabbage
- Pepper, salt, garlic powder, parsley, and curry for preparing

Method:

- Cut the onions and utilize a cooking splash to sauté them in a pot.
- Cut the stem off the green pepper and afterward cut it into equal parts. Reduce the film and the seeds. Make bit size pieces and add to the pot.
- Reduce the leaves of the cabbage, dice it and throw it in the pot.
- Cut the carrots and celery into little pieces and add to the pot
- Cut the mushrooms thickly and add them.

- Add the tomatoes.
- Add garlic powder if you need to.
- Add 12 cups of water; cover the pot and let your soup cook for several hours.

142: Vinegar Dressing

Vinegar dressing can be alluded to as vinaigrettes. For making a vinaigrette presumably the most normal enhanced vinegar which is the white vinegar isn't the ideal sort of vinegar for making a dressing. You can use white wine vinegar. Then again, the sorts and kinds of particularly made vinegar including balsamic, raspberry, or sherry are as various and as shifted it very well maybe

Vinegar dressing has been used to enhance dishes for a ton of years at this point and is the most loved dressing utilized these days by culinary experts to improve dinner or salad that may somehow or another be boring to introduce. The ease of the vinegar is truly what keeps it normal and is broadly used even inside your family cooking.

Ingredients:

- 1 tablespoon white wine vinegar
- 3 tablespoons extra virgin olive oil
- Squeeze genuine salt
- A turn of freshly ground black pepper
- 1-2 tablespoons fresh cleaved spices
- A finely crushed garlic clove
- 2 teaspoons finely cleaved shallots, scallions, or onion
- 2 teaspoons finely crushed or ground ginger

- 2 tablespoons finely ground or disintegrated Parmesan
- 1 teaspoon Dijon mustard
- Spot of squashed red pepper chips
- 1/2 - 1 teaspoon sugar or honey

Method:

- Add the whole of the ingredients to a little bricklayer container, screw on the top, and shake until mixed.
- You can likewise whisk the ingredients together in a bowl or whirr them together in a blender.
- Taste and change flavors whenever wanted.
- Add to salad, prepare, and serve.
- Keep extra dressing in a fixed container in the fridge for 2 - 3 days.

143: Honey Raspberry Vinaigrette

Honey Raspberry Vinaigrette is a sweet recipe. It's an incredible salad dressing for the warm spring and midyear months and adds a brilliant fly of raspberry flavor to any salad recipe. This raspberry dressing is very flexible. However, I love it on my Berry Spinach Salad for an extra increase in raspberry goodness.

Basic, fresh, and modest, the flavors in this custom-made Raspberry Vinaigrette recipe are such a ton better than anything you can purchase at the store! Mix up a clump to keep in your refrigerator to add a sweet and lively kick to all your late spring salad.

Ingredients:

- 2/3 cup balsamic vinegar

- 1 cup fresh raspberries
- 1/4 cup olive oil
- 1 tablespoon white sugar
- 1 tablespoon honey
- 1/2 teaspoon salt

Method:

- Consolidate raspberries and white sugar in a bowl and leave for 10 to 15 minutes until the blend is delicious.
- Crush berries utilizing a fork until condensed (or beat in a blender for 30 seconds if you lean toward dressing to be smoother).
- Fill a glass container with a top then add balsamic vinegar, honey, olive oil, and salt to the container.
- Cover and shake until very much consolidated.

Refrigerate until prepared to utilize.

144: Messy Peppercorn Dressing

Peppercorn dressings are an extraordinary method to introduce particular and remarkable flavors to the bed while giving a sprinkle of splendid tones. A rainbow of hot flavors like white, green, and pink can without much of a stretch make a noteworthy dish. Messy Peppercorn Dressing is a brilliantly smooth dressing with a hot kick from fresh broke peppercorns! It's stunning over salad or utilized as a plunge with vegetable crudités.

Ingredient:

- 1/2 teaspoon salt, or more to taste
- 2 cups plain low-fat yogurt

- 1/4 cup finely chopped green onion
- 1/4 cup ground parmesan cheddar, or more to taste
- 2 tablespoons milk
- 1 tablespoon mayonnaise
- 2 tablespoons finely cut fresh parsley
- 2 teaspoons freshly ground black pepper

Method:

- In a bowl, combine as one yogurt, parmesan cheddar, onion, parsley mayonnaise, ground black pepper, and salt.
- Gradually add and mix in milk until wanted slenderness is accomplished.
- Add more cheddar or salt to change the taste.
- Cover and refrigerate at any rate 1 hour before serving.

A straightforward salad with spinach leaves, mushrooms, and red onion gets deserving of an uncommon event when finished off with older style Sweet Bacon Dressing. So sweet and pungent with huge loads of bacon flavor and a little tang. Thoroughly long for commendable.

Ingredients:

- 1/2 cup white vinegar
- 3 teaspoons corn starch
- 1/4 cup water
- 1/2 teaspoon salt
- 1/2 cups white sugar
- 8 cuts bacon, cooked and disintegrated

Method:

- Whisk together sugar, corn starch, and salt in a medium bowl.
- Gradually mix in vinegar and water, whisking continually.
- Spot disintegrated bacon in a skillet over medium heat then pour sugar blend over bacon.
- Cook and mix continually until the combination thickens.
- Reduce from heat and permit to cool for 10 to 15 minutes before serving.

This Creamy Cilantro Dressing just requires a couple of moments to make and is such a great deal better compared to locally acquired salad dressing. It is incredible on fish, mixed greens, chicken, steak, tacos, vegetables, and then some. It's really simple to make and endures a decent week in the refrigerator. It's flexible and can be utilized as a plunging sauce for veggies and fries, or as a salad dressing, on tacos or barbecued meats, burrito bowls, and on pretty much anything!

Ingredients:

- 2 cloves garlic, squashed
- 1/2 cups mayonnaise
- 2 Anaheim Chile peppers, cooked
- 1/3 cup toasted pumpkin seeds
- 3/4 cup canola oil
- 1/4 cup disintegrated Cotija cheddar
- 1/2 teaspoon salt
- 1/4 cup red wine vinegar
- 1/4 cup water
- 1/4 teaspoon freshly ground black pepper
- 2 packages cilantro, stems reduced

Method:

- Join garlic, mayonnaise, pumpkin seeds, Chile peppers, oil, water, salt, cheddar, and black pepper in a blender or food processor for 1 moment or until smooth.

- Add cilantro in groups, beating for around 40 seconds for each clump.
- Pour combination in a glass bowl.
- Cover and refrigerate for 1 hour before serving.

147: Simple Sweet and Spicy Salad Dressing

This Spicy Sweet Salad Dressing Recipe is a basic vinaigrette made with only 5 ingredients. It requires 5 minutes to make and is amazing to dress an assortment of salads. It's so totally sweet and fiery and is a simple method to light up your ordinary salad.

Ingredients:

- 1 cup vegetable oil
- 1 cup crushed onion
- 3/4 cup white sugar
- 1/4 cup apple juice vinegar
- 1/3 cup ketchup
- 1 tablespoon Worcestershire sauce

Method:

- Mix onion, ketchup, sugar, apple juice vinegar, and Worcestershire sauce in a bowl until sugar has broken down.
- Cautiously mix in vegetable oil until completely consolidated.
- Cover and refrigerate for 60 minutes.
- Mix before serving.

Celery and apples share a ton for all intents and purpose; they're fresh, succulent, and delightful wellsprings of dietary fiber and vitamin C. Yet, it's the manners by which they contrast that makes them a particularly novel and free combo.

Ingredients:

- 1/2 stick of spread or margarine
- 1/2 tsp of crushed garlic (optional)
- 1 medium onion, cut fine
- 1 tsp dried sage
- 4 - 6 celery ribs, washed and cut fine
- 1 tsp dried thyme
- 1 sweet apple (any assortment) stripped, cored, and cut fine
- 1/2 cup chicken stock or stock
- around 8 ounces of dried breadcrumbs or stuffing blocks

Method:

- Dissolve the spread in a big skillet and sauté the onion and garlic over low heat until just mollified.
- Add the celery and apples; blend well and keep on sauting for a few minutes, until all ingredients are covered and are starting to mollify.
- Add the breadcrumbs or stuffing 3D squares and throw them in the container to cover, then add the stock and keep on cooking for around three minutes, or until the

fluid is very much assimilated and the pieces or 3D shapes are soaked.

If you are searching for something luscious yet sound and wellness agreeable, go for the Greek salad unquestionably. Greek salad is a scrumptious summer dish that started in Greece. It is likewise called 'summer salad' in certain nations however locals call it horiatiki Salata, 'country salad,' or 'town salad,' which fundamental ingredients incorporate delicious tomatoes, cucumbers, green chime pepper or yellow ringer pepper, cubed feta cheddar, red onion, and Kalamata olives, with salt, dried oregano, and olive oil flavors. A few however incorporate vinegar, berries of escapades, lemon juice, and parsley to add taste.

Ingredients:

- Dried oregano - 1/2 tsp
- Ocean salt - 1/4 tsp ocean salt
- Clove garlic - 1 piece, crushed
- Extra virgin olive oil - 3 tablespoons
- Black pepper - 1/4 teaspoon
- Cucumber cut into thick parts
- Tomatoes cut into wedges
- Onion rings
- Sweet yellow pepper, in lumps
- Basil leaves (optional)
- Feta cheddar - around 120 grams, cubed
- Green ringer pepper, julienned
- Lemon juice - 1/2 tablespoons (optional)

- Kalamata olives

Method:

- To start with, you blend olive oil, garlic, lemon juice, salt, pepper, and oregano.
- Then, you blend every one of the vegetables in a single bowl and add the dressing.
- Present with black pepper to finish.

150: Tomato Mozzarella Salad

Look at this extraordinary-looking and incredible tasting dish! Since this tomato mozzarella salad has red tomatoes, white mozzarella, and green basil, the tones look extraordinary together, and the dish tastes incredible as well. The blend of fresh mozzarella cheddar, red tomatoes, and green basil makes this dish extraordinary to take a gander at, and it makes the salad scrumptious! Besides, when you are adding a spice like basil, which adds a green tone, you will make the salad much more delicious and surprisingly more beautiful.

This tomato salad is not difficult to make. Simply consolidate chopped tomatoes, fresh mozzarella cheddar, and basil. Utilize a touch of olive oil and balsamic vinegar to gently dress this salad. Or then again, avoid the vinegar and simply utilize olive oil to dress it - it will in any case be exceptionally delectable.

Ingredients:

- 1/2 little white onion, cubed little
- 3 cups sweet grape, cherry, or bigger cleaved tomatoes

- 2/3 cup little cubed mozzarella cheddar
- 2/3 tablespoon balsamic vinegar (great quality)
- 1 tablespoon extra-virgin olive oil (great quality)
- 4 leaves of romaine lettuce (measured to suit the size of servings you need)
- Italian parsley for decorate
- Salt and pepper to taste

Method:

- Blend the above ingredients in a bowl.
- Mix the olive oil and vinegar in a cup by beating them along with a fork.
- Blend this in well with the tomato combination.
- Season the blend with pepper and salt (according to taste).
- Spoon the tomato combination into an appealing heap on top of the lettuce and trimming with parsley.
- Serve this immediately...you don't need your lettuce to get unstable.
- Enjoy!

151: Cobb Salad

This is quite possibly the most loved salad arrangement of people across the world. With every one of the ingredients like eggs, bacon, chickens, and salad dressing, it simply tastes marvelous! Go through this basic recipe given underneath. It requires just 50 minutes to finish and serve the salad at your table.

Ingredients:

- Three eggs
- 8 cuts of bacon
- 1 head destroyed ice shelf lettuce
- Two cultivated and cut tomatoes
- 3 cups chicken meat (cut, cooked)
- disintegrated blue cheddar - 3/4 cup
- 1 stripped, pitted, and cubed avocado
- Farm style salad dressing - 1 (8 ounce) bottle
- 3 chopped green onions

Method:

- Put eggs in a skillet and with cold water cover the eggs.
- Allow the water to bubble. Put a cover, reduce it from heat, and let the eggs stay in the hot water for around 10 to 12 minutes.
- Take the eggs out from the boiling water, cool them down, strip and afterward hack them.
- Spot the cuts of bacon in a major, profound skillet.
- Cook the bacon cuts on medium-high heat until every one of the cuts is consistently earthy colored on all sides.
- Strain, disintegrate the pieces, and put away the pieces.
- Separate the destroyed lettuce in the various plates similarly.
- Similarly gap and spot bacon, chicken, tomatoes, blue cheddar, eggs, green onions, and avocado in a line on top of the chunk of ice lettuce leaves.
- Sprinkle with Ranch-style salad dressing as per your necessities and enjoy the salad.

- You can utilize feta cheddar rather than blue cheddar.
- You can embellish it with cheddar and bubbled corn.
- You can add vegetables like carrots, zucchini, yellow squash, cabbages, and so forth to make it nutritious.
- You can likewise add mayonnaise if you need to make a rich surface.
- You can likewise utilize serve this salad with singed chicken wings.

152: Shrimp and Avocado Salad

This is a stunning salad recipe that is incredible as a side salad or as a light lunch meeting recipe. Serve it in lettuce cups for lunch alongside some fresh hard bread and an extraordinary treat. Simply awesome!

Ingredients:

- 1 avocado
- 1 cup celery, meagerly cut
- 2 tablespoons Italian salad dressing
- salt and pepper to taste
- 4 tablespoons mayonnaise
- 2 teaspoons lemon juice
- 1 pound frozen cooked shrimp, defrosted

Method:

- Join the shrimp, celery, Italian dressing, and mayonnaise.
- Season to taste with salt and pepper.
- Chill, covered until prepared to serve.
- When prepared to serve, strip and dice the avocado.

- Blend promptly with the lemon juice to keep the avocado from going dull.
- Add to the shrimp combination and blend delicately.

This recipe is scrumptious, however quite simple. It's an extraordinary recipe to serve the organization at a grill since it stretches made beyond and sits in the cooler for a couple of hours until you are prepared for it. The best summer engaging plans do not need the host and entertainer to be in the kitchen cooking while visitors relax outside.

Ingredients:

- 1/4 cups red wine vinegar
- 3 huge cucumbers, stripped and meagerly cut
- 1/2 teaspoon celery salt
- 1 tablespoon honey
- 1/2 head of lettuce, destroyed
- a great squeeze of black pepper
- 4 tablespoons olive oil
- 1/2 teaspoon fresh dill, cleaved
- 1 teaspoon Dijon mustard

Method:

- Prepare every one of the ingredients completely in a huge salad bowl.
- Chill for 2 hours before serving.

154: Lime Jello Cottage Cheese Salad

This is an exquisite light salad recipe that is ideal for a late spring grill yet functions admirably throughout the year on a smorgasbord table. The expansion of curds may sound odd; however, it is an extraordinary flavor that blends in with the Jello. The mash of the celery and green pepper add another layer of flavor and fresh taste.

Ingredients:

- 1 cup bubbling water
- 1 - 3-ounce package lime jam powder
- 1/2 cup cold water
- 1/2 cup mayonnaise
- salt and pepper
- 1 teaspoon vinegar or lemon juice
- 3/4 cup cleaved celery
- 1/2 green pepper, cleaved
- 1/2 onion, cleaved

Method:

- Mix with mixer and chill until firm 1" from the edge of the dish.
- Transform it into a bowl and beat it until it turns out to be light and fleecy.
- Overlap in 1 cup curds, celery, onion, and green pepper.
- Chill completely before serving.

155: Pork Chops

Searching for various approaches to fix pork hacks? Eating them seared is delectable and filling however there are numerous alternative ways that they can be readied that will draw out the very scrumptious flavor that you love. Attempt

Pork Chops basic and delectable recipe for a scrumptious option in contrast to ordinary searing. Pork hacks can be utilized to make astonishing meals that too consistently. These are the simplest dishes that one can make at home. The plans for pork slashes are not muddled and fabulous plans can be made with them.

Ingredients:

- 1/3 cup bourbon
- 1 tsp black pepper
- 1/3 cup soy sauce (low sodium)
- 2 tbsp. juice vinegar
- 3 cloves garlic
- 3 tbsp. Brown sugar
- 1 tsp red pepper pieces
- 1 tbsp. cornstarch

Method:

- Combine the initial seven ingredients as one.
- Save ¼ cup of the blend.
- Pour the leftover marinade over the pork hacks in a fixed plastic sack.
- Refrigerate the pork hacks for the time being.
- Before flame broiling the cleaves, blend cornstarch into the ¼ cup of unused marinade.
- Tenderly heat until effervescent and thickened into a brilliant sauce.
- Serve the grilled pork cleaves with a spoonful of the sauce over the top.

Bean salad is consistently a success at summer grills and family social affairs. They are not difficult to plan, modest to make, and make an extraordinary backup to any feast. Attempt this Hot Green Bean Salad with Potatoes recipe at your next family gathering. Your family will make certain to adore it.

Ingredients:

- 2 tbsp. olive oil
- 1 cut onion finely cut
- 1 little or ½ medium onion, chopped
- 1/8 tsp salt
- 2 tbsp. corn starch
- 1/8 tsp black pepper
- 1 to 1 ¼ cup sugar
- 1 cup white vinegar
- 2 to 4 medium potatoes, cubed and cooked
- 32 oz. Green beans, cooked
- 4 cuts of bacon, disintegrated

Method:

- Cut bacon into little pieces with kitchen shears.
- Fry the bacon until firm.
- Spot the bacon on a paper towel to deplete the bacon fat.
- In a spotless profound fry, the dish adds olive oil, little cleaved onion, salt, and pepper.
- Cook over medium heat until the onion has a marginally brilliant shading.
- Keep cooking the onion and add the corn starch and blend into the onion completely.
- Add the sugar and blend once more.
- Add the vinegar to the whole blend and continue to mix over the heat until every one of the ingredients has merged.
- Permit the combination to cook until hot and effervescent. When the sauce has thickened, reduce the heat.
- Cook the green beans and potatoes together until both are delicate.
- Flush and channel in a colander.
- Spot the beans and potatoes into a serving dish.
- Pour the warm sauce on the potatoes & beans.
- Sprinkle the finely cleaved onion on top alongside the firm bacon bits.

Spinach and Cranberry Salad are wonderful! It's a fast and simple salad you can gather in around ten to fifteen minutes. What's more, that incorporates making the dressing! It just uses a modest bunch of ingredients making the simplicity of planning extremely basic. This delicious salad incorporates spinach, red onion, goat cheddar, almonds, and dried cranberries.

Ingredients:

- 1 cup dried cranberries
- 1 lb. spinach, flushed and attacked pieces
- 2 tbsp. crushed onion
- 1 tbsp. margarine
- 3/4 cup almonds, whitened and fragmented
- 2 tbsp. toasted sesame seeds
- 1/4 tbsp. paprika
- 1 tbsp. poppy seeds
- 1/2 cup white sugar
- 1/4 cup white wine vinegar
- 1/2 cup vegetable oil
- 1/4 cup juice vinegar

Method:

- Heat a little skillet at medium heat and liquefy the margarine.
- Add the almonds and cook until toasted. Permit the almonds to cool.

- In a huge bowl, combine as one the cranberries, spinach, and almonds.
- In a different bowl, whisk together the sugar, vegetable oil, white wine vinegar, juice vinegar, onion, poppy seeds, paprika, and sesame seeds.
- Not long before serving, throw the spinach in the dressing blend.

158: Broccoli Salad with a Twist

Most Broccoli Salads have Mayonnaise as the essential ingredient. However, this Salad utilizes Cream Cheese which adds a decent flavor and the apple juice gives it a truly fun zip. Likewise, the calorie distinction is insane. For the Mayonnaise salad, there are around 1495 calories. This Easy Salad utilizes Cream Cheese, which slices the calories to 776!!!! Fundamentally, for 6 servings this salad (without the bacon!) is 129 calories for each serving contrasted with 250 calories for the mayonnaise.

Ingredients:

- 1/3 cup mandarin oranges
- 3 tbsp. mayonnaise
- 1/2 cups fresh broccoli florets
- 4 bacon strips, cooked and chopped
- 1/4 cup finely cleaved onion
- 1 tbsp. sugar
- 3/4 cup destroyed cheddar
- 2 tbsp. white vinegar

Method:

- In a big bowl combine as one the broccoli, bacon, onion, and cheddar.
- In a different bowl, join the mayo, sugar, and vinegar- blend well.
- Pour the sauce over the broccoli combination and combine as one.
- Cover with saran wrap and refrigerate for at least 60 minutes.
- Not long before serving, sprinkle chilled mandarin oranges over the top.

159: Pear and Pecan Salad

Simple to prepare ahead, this spinach salad is loaded up with sweet cooked pears, smooth walnuts, tart goat cheddar, crunchy pomegranates with a simple hand-crafted balsamic dressing is an ideal occasion side dish or a scrumptious fall meal. This Roasted Pear Salad is a recipe you will be eager to set aside a few minutes and time once more.

Ingredients:

- 1/3 cup Italian salad dressing
- 1 pack Italian salad
- 1/2 cup walnut parts
- 1/2 cup destroyed mozzarella cheddar
- 1 pear (stripped, cored, and cubed)

Method:

- Throw all ingredients (aside from dressing) in a bowl.

- When prepared to serve, sprinkle a touch of Italian dressing over the blend and throw well to guarantee an in any event, covering.
- Topping with lemon or mandarin oranges.

160: Pistachio Fruit Salad

Making this pistachio salad is speedy, simple, and modest. It doesn't make any difference if you call it Watergate salad, pistachio cushion, or pistachio fruit salad, they're all names for a similar delightful pastry. Any gathering is an incredible chance to prepare a cluster of this pistachio salad. I realize I continue to call this a salad when it is more similar to a sweet.

Ingredients:

- 1 package moment without sugar pistachio pudding blend
- 1 cup decreased fat whipped besting
- 1 can fruit mixed drink, depleted
- 1 can mandarin oranges, depleted
- 1/4 cup maraschino cherries
- 1 can squashed pineapple
- A modest bunch of small scale marshmallows

Method:

- Channel the pineapple juice into a huge bowl.
- Rush in the pudding blend for around two minutes.
- Add pineapple, fruit mixed drink, oranges, cherries, and marshmallows.
- Cautiously crease in the whipped garnish to keep it fleecy.

- Cover with saran wrap and refrigerate until serving.

Figure out how to cook extraordinary Chicken with ginger pesto. Crecipe.com conveys the fine determination of value Chicken with ginger pesto plans furnished with appraisals, audits, and blending tips. Get one of our Chicken with ginger pesto recipes and plan a delightful and solid treat for your family or companions. Great hunger.

Ingredients:

- 2 cloves garlic, crushed
- 1 kg. boneless and skinless chicken bosom parts
- 1 pack green onions, cut into 1/4-inch pieces
- 1/4 cup vegetable oil
- 1/2 cup dry white wine
- 2 tablespoons ground fresh ginger root
- 1 teaspoon white sugar
- 1 tablespoon salt

Method:

- In a medium pot, pour 2-3 cups of softly salted water then add chicken bosoms.
- Heat to the point of boiling, lower heat, and stew for 8-10 minutes or until cooked through.
- Permit chicken to cool in the stock.
- When cool, reduce from stock and put away.
- Heat vegetable oil in a different skillet over medium-high heat then mix in garlic, ginger, salt, and sugar.

- Lower heat and cook for 15-20 minutes or until garlic is delicate.
- Mix in onions and cook for 10 minutes more until onions are delicate.
- Cut chicken bosoms daintily, orchestrate on a plate then top with the ginger combination.

162: Ginger-Glazed Salmon

A marginally sweet, yet zesty and unimaginably tasty ginger coat makes this overpowering salmon recipe that is easy to get ready and meets up in a short time. This recipe is easy to make, yet great. The marinade gives the fish a sweet taste that my family goes crazy for! If it's excessively cold out to barbecue it, you likewise may cook it. Get the flakey salmon surface you've generally needed with a delightful maple ginger sauce for sure.

Ingredients:

- 1 tablespoon Dijon mustard
- 1/2 kg. salmon filets
- 1 tablespoon honey
- 2 teaspoons olive oil
- 2 teaspoons ground fresh ginger

Method:

- Join Dijon mustard, honey, ginger, and olive oil in a little bowl.
- Spot salmon filets in a preparing dish and equally brush with the blend.

- Prepare in a pre-warmed broiler (350 degrees F) for 15-20 minutes.

Most food sources taste better when blended in with the appropriate enhancing or dressing. Be it a fundamental dish or, a canapé, nothing beats a decent food with a similarly decent dressing. A common steak gets professional when presented with a flavorsome sauce. Fruits like strawberry work better with plunges like whipped cream or chocolate.

Make a cluster of this toward the end of the week and enjoy fresh salads throughout the week (truly, simply toss this on some child spinach, and the writing is on the wall! A salad!), or utilize some as a marinade for grilled chicken or veggies. It will remain fresh in the refrigerator for a month, leaving you a lot of time to go through it.

Ingredients:

- 3 cloves garlic, crushed
- 1 lemon, squeezed
- 1 cup olive oil
- Ground black pepper to taste
- 3 tablespoons crushed fresh ginger root
- 1/4 cup soy sauce
- 2 teaspoons honey
- 1 teaspoon arranged mustard (Dijon-style)

Method:

- Combine as one lemon juice, ginger, garlic, honey, mustard, and black pepper in a medium bowl until altogether consolidated.
- Mix in olive oil gradually and blend until joined with different ingredients.

Store in a glass compartment and refrigerate until prepared for serving.

164: Tropical Ginger Shrimp

This Tropical Ginger Shrimp finished off with shrimp and a fruit salsa is a finished meal. Big bits of ginger-soy marinated shrimp and tropical fruit salsa with mango, pineapple, kiwifruit, and mandarin oranges are delicately thrown with child spinach leaves and long strands of pasta in this tropical-enlivened dish.

Ingredients:

- Sticks
- 1 onion, cut
- 1/4 kind sized shrimp, stripped and deveined
- 2 cloves garlic, stripped
- 1/4 cup lemon juice
- 1/2 cup olive oil
- 2 tablespoons ground fresh ginger root
- 2 tablespoons crushed cilantro leaves
- 1 teaspoon paprika
- 1/2 teaspoon salt
- 2 teaspoons sesame oil
- 1/2 teaspoon ground black pepper

Method:

- Consolidate onion, lemon juice, garlic, olive oil, ginger, sesame oil, cilantro, paprika, salt, and pepper in a blender and puree until smooth.
- Save a limited quantity for treating.
- Pour the combination into a big bowl and add shrimp.
- Coat shrimp with blend, cover, and refrigerate for at any rate 2 hours.
- When prepared, dispose of abundance marinade and string shrimp onto sticks.
- Cook in a pre-warmed flame broil over medium-high heat for 2 minutes for every side or until shrimp is cooked through.
- Brush with marinade while cooking.

Conclusion:

Fasting is an extraordinary method to keep the body and psyche solid and clean. Numerous people that training Intermittent fasting consistently guarantee they've taken in a ton about their dietary patterns also. The explanation is because they have a great deal of time to consider food and which food sources they're wanting on their fasting days.

The degree of adrenaline your body produces is likewise expanded during momentary fasting, which places your body's capacity to consume fat into overdrive and work twice as hard. Join this with your expanded digestion and you can perceive how shedding pounds would be so basic with Intermittent fasting.

Intermittent fasting isn't prudent for all people. This is just useful for people without medical issues. Whenever you want to try intermittent fasting, you should counsel first with your doctor before you push through.

KETO DIET FOR WOMEN OVER 50

The Complete Ketogenic Diet Step by Step To Learn How to Easily Lose Weight for Woman

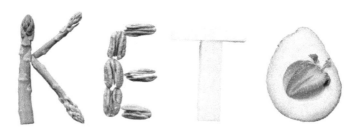

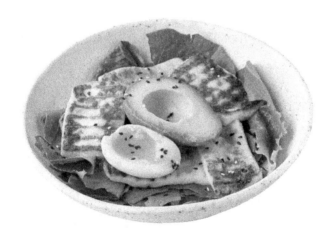

information is without a contract or any type of guarantee assurance.

The trademarks used are without any consent, and the publication of the trademark is without permission or backing by the trademark owner. All trademarks and brands within this book are for clarifying purposes only and are owned by the owners themselves, not affiliated with this document.

Introduction

The keto diet is a diet that has higher and lower fat values. It decreases glucose & insulin levels and changes the body's digestion away from carbohydrates and more towards fat & ketones. A word used in a low-carb diet is "Ketogenic." The concept is to provide more calories from fat and protein and few from sugars. The consumption of a high, low-sugar diet, adequate-protein, is used in medicine to achieve difficult (unstable) epilepsy control in young people. Instead of sugar, the diet allows the body to eat fats. Usually, the nutritious starches are converted to sugar, which will then be distributed throughout the body and is particularly important in filling the mind's work. Keto diet can cause enormous declines in the levels of glucose and insulin.

How food affects your body

Our metabolic procedures survive if we do not get the right details, and our well-being declines. We can get overweight, malnourished, and at risk for the worsening of diseases and disorders, such as inflammatory disease, diabetes, and cardiovascular disease if women get an unhealthy amount of essential nutrients or nourishment that provides their body with inadequate guidance. The dietary supplements allow the cells in our bodies to serve their essential capacities. This quote from a well-known workbook shows how dietary supplements are important for our physical work. Supplements are the nourishment feed substances necessary for the growth, development, and support of the body's capacities. Fundamental claimed that when a supplement is absent, capability sections and thus decrease in human health. The metabolic processes are delayed when the intake of supplements usually may not fulfill the cell activity's supplement requirements.

The keto diet involves keeping to a relatively low-carb, high-fat diet to put the body into a physiological state called ketosis. This makes fat intake increasingly productive for the health. When starting the diet, the ketogenic diet can induce a decrease in the drive, as the dieter will suffer side effects of carb removal and possibly low carb influenza. Whenever the detox and influenza-like symptoms have gone, and the dieter has transitioned to the reduced way of living, leading to weight loss from the diet, the charisma would in all likelihood reset and probably be comparable to earlier. Although the drive alert has a lot of credibility in the mainstream, in other words, supplementation provides advice to our bodies on how to function. In this sense, nourishment can be seen as a source of "information for the body." Pondering food along these lines gives one a view of the nourishment beyond calories or grams, fantastic food sources, or bad food sources. Instead of avoiding food sources, this perspective pushes us to reflect on the nutrients we can add. Instead of reviewing nourishment as the enemy, we look at nourishment to reduce health and disease by having the body look after ability.

Kidney and Heart Disease

When the body is low in electrolytes and fluid over the increased pee, electrolyte loss, such as magnesium, sodium, and potassium, can be caused. This will render people inclined to suffer serious kidney problems. Flushing out is not a joke and can lead to light-headedness, damage to the kidney, or kidney problems. Just like electrolytes are essential for the heart's standard stomping, this can place a dieter at the risk of cardiac arrhythmia. "Electrolyte appears to lack are not joking, and that may bring in an irregular heartbeat, that can be harmful,"

Yo-yo Dieting designs

When individuals encounter difficulties staying on the prohibitive diet indefinitely, the keto diet will also cause yo-yo dieting. That can have other adverse effects on the body.

Other effects

Other responses can involve terrible breath, fatigue, obstruction, irregular menstrual periods, reduced bone density, and trouble with rest. For even the most part, other consequences are not so much considered since it is impossible to observe dieters on a long-term assumption to discover the food schedule's permanent effects.

Wholesome Concerns

"There is still a dread amongst healthcare professionals that certain high intakes of extremely unhealthy fats will have a longer journey negative effect," she explained. Weight loss will also, for the time being, complicate the data. As overweight people get in form, paying less attention to how they do so, they sometimes end up with much better lipid profiles and blood glucose levels.

In comparison, the keto diet is extremely low in particular natural ingredients, fruits, nuts, and veggies that are as nutritious as a whole. Without these supplements, fiber, some carbohydrates, minerals, including phytochemicals that come along with these nourishments, will move through people on a diet. In the long run, this has vital public health consequences, such as bone degradation and increased risk of infinite diseases.

Sodium

The mixture of sodium (salt), fat, sugar, including bunches of sodium, will make inexpensive food more delicious for many people. However, diets rich in sodium will trigger fluid retention, which is why you can feel puffy, bloated, or swelled up in the aftermath of consuming cheap food. For those with pulse problems, a diet rich in sodium is also harmful. Sodium can increase circulatory stress and add weight to the cardiovascular structure. If one survey reveals, about % of grown-ups lose how much salt is in their affordable food meals. The study looked at 993 adults and found that the initial prediction was often smaller than the actual figure (1,292 mg). This suggests the sodium gauges in the abundance of 1,000 mg is off. One affordable meal could be worth a significant proportion of your day.

Impact on the Respiratory Framework

An overabundance of calories can contribute to weight gain from cheap foods. This will add to the weight. Obesity creates the risk of respiratory conditions, including asthma with shortness of breath. The extra pounds can put pressure on the heart and lungs, and with little intervention, side effects can occur. When you walk, climb stairs, or work out, you can notice trouble breathing. For youngsters, the possibility of respiratory problems is especially obvious. One research showed that young people who consume cheap food at least three days a week are bound to develop asthma.

Impact on the focal sensory system

For the time being, cheap food may satisfy hunger; however, long-haul effects are more detrimental. Individuals who consume inexpensive food and processed bakery items are 51 percent bound to generate depression than people who do not eat or eat either of those foods.

Impact on the conceptive framework

The fixings in cheap food and lousy nourishment can affect your money. One analysis showed that phthalates are present in prepared nourishment. Phthalates are synthetic compounds that can mess with the way your body's hormones function. Introduction to substantial amounts of these synthetics, like birth absconds, could prompt regenerative problems.

Impact on the integumentary framework (skin, hair, nails)

The food you eat may affect your skin's appearance, but it's not going to be the food you imagine. The responsibility for skin dry out breakouts has traditionally been claimed by sweets and sticky nourishments such as pizza. Nevertheless, as per the Mayo Clinic, there are starches. Carb-rich foods cause glucose jumps, and these sudden leaps in glucose levels can induce inflammation of the skin. Additionally, as shown by one investigation, young people and young women who consume inexpensive food at any pace three days a week are expected to create skin inflammation. Dermatitis is a skin disease that causes dry, irritated skin spots that are exacerbated.

Impact on the skeletal framework (bones)

Acids in the mouth can be enlarged by carbohydrates and sugar in inexpensive food and treated food. These acids may distinguish tooth lacquer. Microorganisms can take hold when the tooth veneer disappears, and depressions can occur. Weight will also prompt issues with bone thickness and bulk. The more severe chance of falling and breaking bones is for heavy individuals. It is important to continue training, develop muscles that support the bones, and sustain a balanced diet to prevent bone loss. One investigation showed that the measure of calories, sugar, and sodium in cheap food meals remains, to a large degree, constant because of attempts to bring problems to light and make women more intelligent consumers. As women get busier and eat out more often, it could have antagonistic effects on women and America's healthcare structure.

Chapter 1: Keto Diet and Its Benefits

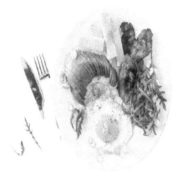

In the case of a ketogenic diet, the aim is to restrict carbohydrate intake to break down fat for power. When this occurs, to produce ketones that are by-products of the metabolism, the liver breaks down fat. These ketones are used in the absence of glucose to heat the body. A ketogenic diet takes the body into a "ketosis" mode. A metabolic condition that happens as ketone bodies in the blood contains most of the body's energy rather than glucose from carbohydrate-produced foods (such as grains, all sources of sugar or fruit). This compares with a glycolytic disorder, where blood glucose produces most of the body's power.

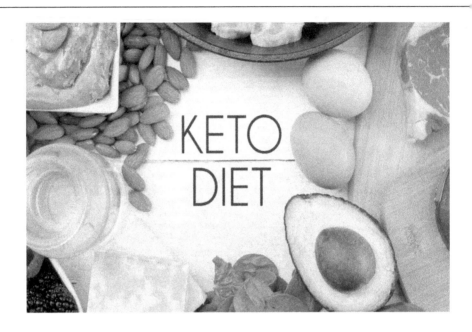

1.1. Keto Diet and its Success

The keto diet is successful in many studies, especially among obese men and women. The results suggest that KD can help manage situations such as:

- Obesity.
- Heart disease.

It is difficult to relate the ketogenic diet to cardiovascular disease risk factors. Several studies have shown that keto diets may contribute to substantial reductions in overall cholesterol, rises in levels of HDL cholesterol, decreases in levels of triglycerides and decreases in levels of LDL cholesterol, as well as possible changes in levels of blood pressure.

- Neurological disorders, including Alzheimer's, dementia, multiple sclerosis and Parkinson's.
- Polycystic ovarian syndrome (PCOS), among women of reproductive age, is the most prevalent endocrine condition.
- Certain forms of cancer, including cancers of the liver, colon, pancreas and ovaries.
- Diabetes Type 2. Among type 2 diabetics, it can also minimize the need for drugs.
- Seizure symptoms and seizures.
- And others.

1.2. Why Do the Ketogenic Diet

By exhausting the body from its sugar store, Ketogenic works to start sorting fat and protein for vitality, inducing ketosis (and weight loss).

1. Helps in weight loss

To convert fat into vitality, it takes more effort than it takes to turn carbohydrates into vitality. A ketogenic diet along these lines can help speed up weight loss. In comparison, because the diet is rich in protein, it doesn't leave you starving as most diets do. Five findings uncovered tremendous weight loss from a ketogenic diet in a meta-examination of 13 complex randomized controlled preliminaries.

2. Diminishes skin break out

There are different causes for the breakout of the skin, and food and glucose can be established. Eating a balanced diet of prepared and refined sugars can alter gut microorganisms and emphasize sensational variances in glucose, both of which would affect the skin's health. Therefore, that is anything but surprising that a keto diet may reduce a few instances of skin inflammation by decreasing carb entry.

3. May help diminish the danger of malignancy

There has been a lot of study on the ketogenic diet and how it could effectively forestall or even cure those malignant growths. One investigation showed that the ketogenic diet might be a corresponding effective treatment with chemotherapy and radiation in people with malignancy. It is because it can cause more oxidative concern than in ordinary cells in malignancy cells.

Some hypotheses indicate that it may decrease insulin entanglements, which could be linked to some cancers because the ketogenic diet lowers elevated glucose.

4. Improves heart health

There is some indication that the diet will boost cardiac health by lowering cholesterol by accessing the ketogenic diet in a balanced manner (which looks at avocados as a healthy fat rather than pork skins). One research showed that LDL ("Terrible") cholesterol levels fundamentally expanded among those adopting the keto diet. In turn, the LDL ("terrible") cholesterol fell.

5. May secure mind working

More study into the ketogenic diet and even the mind is needed. A few studies indicate that the keto diet has Neuro-protective effects. These can help treat or curtail Parkinson's, Alzheimer's, and even some rest problems. One research also showed that young people had increased and psychological work during a ketogenic diet.

6. Possibly lessens seizures

The theory that the combination of fat, protein, and carbohydrates modifies how vitality is utilized by the body, inducing ketosis. Ketosis is an abnormal level of Ketone in the blood. In people with epilepsy, ketosis will prompt a reduction in seizures.

7. Improves health in women with PCOS

An endocrine condition that induces augmented ovaries with pimples is polycystic ovarian disorder PCOS). On the opposite, a high-sugar diet can affect those with PCOS. On the ketogenic diet and PCOS, there are not many clinical tests. One pilot study involving five women on 24 weeks showed that the ketogenic diet:

- Aided hormone balance
- Improved luteinizing hormone (ILH)/follicle-invigorating hormone (FSH) proportions
- Increased weight loss
- Improved fasting insulin

For children who suffer the adverse effects of a particular problem (such as Lennox-gastaut disease or Rett disorder) and do not respond to seizure prescription, keto is also prescribed as suggested by the epilepsy foundation.

They note that the number of seizures these children had can be greatly reduced by keto, with 10 to 15 percent turns out to be sans seizure. It may also help patients to reduce the portion of their prescription in some circumstances. Be it as it can, the ketogenic diet still many effective trials to back up its advantages. For adults with epilepsy, the keto diet can likewise be helpful. It was considered as preferable to other diets in supporting people with:

- Epilepsy
- Type 2 diabetes
- Type 1 diabetes
- High blood pressure
- Heart disease
- Polycystic ovary syndrome
- Fatty liver disease
- Cancer
- Migraines

- Alzheimer's infection
- Parkinson's infection
- Chronic inflammation
- High blood sugar levels
- Obesity

The ketogenic diet will be beneficial, regardless of whether you are not in danger from any of these disorders. A portion of the advantages that are enjoyed by the vast majority are:

- An increment in vitality
- Improved body arrangement
- Better cerebrum work
- A decline in aggravation

As should be clear, the ketogenic diet has a vast variety of advantages, but is it preferable to other diets?

8. Treating epilepsy — the origins of the ketogenic diet

Until sometime in 1998, the major analysis on epilepsy and the keto diets was not distributed. Of about 150 children, almost each of whom had several seizures a week, despite taking two psychosis drugs in either situation. The children were given a one-year initial ketogenic diet. Around 34 percent of infants, or slightly more than 33 percent, had a 90 percent decline in seizures after three months.

The healthy diet was claimed to be "more feasible than just a substantial lot of new anticonvulsant medications and is much endured by families and kids when it is effective." Not only was the keto diet supportive. It was, however, more useful than other drugs usually used.

9. Improving blood pressure with the ketogenic diet

A low-sugar intake is more effective at reducing the pulse than just a low-fat or moderate-fat diet. Restricting starches often provides preferable results over the mix of a low-fat regimen and a relaxing weight-loss/pulse.

10. The power to improve Alzheimer's disease

Alzheimer's disease patients also agree with organic chemistry." high sugar acceptance deepens academic performance in patient populations with Alzheimer's infectious disease." It means that more starches are consumed in the cerebrum. Will the reverse (trying to eat fewer carbs) improve the functioning of the cerebrum?

Other mental health benefits that ketone bodies have:

- They forestall neuronal loss.
- They ensure synapses against various sorts of damage.
- They save neuron work.

•

1.3. The Benefits of Ketogenic Diet

The board provides many substantial advantages when choosing a ketogenic diet for diabetes. Living in a stable ketosis state causes a tremendous change in blood glucose regulation and weight loss. Other frequent advantages provided include:

- Improvements in insulin affectability
- Lower circulatory strain
- Usually enhancements in cholesterol levels.
- Reduced reliance on taking drugs

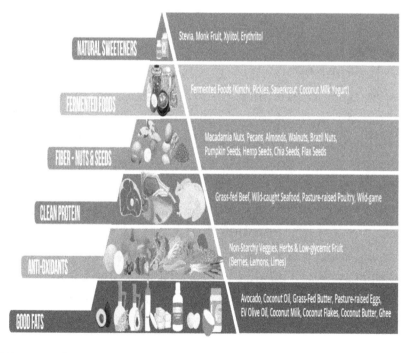

NATURAL SWEETENERS	Stevia, Monk Fruit, Xylitol, Erythritol
FERMENTED FOODS	Fermented Foods (Kimchi, Pickles, Sauerkraut, Coconut Milk Yogurt)
FIBER - NUTS & SEEDS	Macadamia Nuts, Pecans, Almonds, Walnuts, Brazil Nuts, Pumpkin Seeds, Hemp Seeds, Chia Seeds, Flax Seeds
CLEAN PROTEIN	Grass-fed Beef, Wild-caught Seafood, Pasture-raised Poultry, Wild-game
ANTI-OXIDANTS	Non-Starchy Veggies, Herbs & Low-glycemic Fruit (Berries, Lemons, Limes)
GOOD FATS	Avocado, Coconut Oil, Grass-Fed Butter, Pasture-raised Eggs, EV Olive Oil, Coconut Milk, Coconut Flakes, Coconut Butter, Ghee

We send you a short science behind the ketogenic diet in this book and how it attempts to give these particular benefits.

1. Weight loss and support

The ketogenic diet's significant benefit is achieving accelerated weight loss, reducing starches necessary to be in a ketosis state, causing both a noteworthy decrease in muscle vs. fats and bulk increase and maintenance. Studies have shown that a low-carb, keto diet can produce an all-inclusive duration of solid weight loss. For one year, a big person had the opportunity to lose, by and large, 15 kilograms. It was 3 kg, which is more than the low-fat food used in the study carried out.

2. Blood glucose control

The other main reason for maintaining a ketogenic diet for people with diabetes is its ability to reduce and regulate glucose levels. The substitute (macronutrient) that improves glucose the most is starch. Since the keto diet is low in starch, the greater rises in glucose are dispensed with. Ketogenic diets prove that they are effective in reducing hba1c, a long-term blood glucose regulation percentage. A natural decrease of 17 mmol/mol (1.5 percent) in hba1c levels for persons with type 2 diabetes. People with other forms of diabetes, such as diabetes and LADA, can also expect to see a strong decline in glucose levels and increase control. Remember that if an increase in blood glucose regulation is sustained over different years, this will reduce intricacies. It is necessary to play it safe for those on insulin, or otherwise at risk of hypos, to avoid the incidence of hypos.

Decreasing drug reliance on diabetes. Since it is so effective at lowering glucose levels, the keto diet provides the added benefit of allowing people with type 2 diabetes to decrease their dependency on diabetes medication.

Persons on insulin and other hypertension prescriptions (Sulphonylureas & Glinides, for example) may need to reduce their portions before initiating a ketogenic diet to avoid hypotension. For advice on this, contact your primary care provider.

3. Insulin affectability

To further restore insulin affectability, a ketogenic diet has emerged since it dispenses with the root driver of insulin obstruction, which is too high insulin levels in the bloodstream. This diet advances supported periods with low insulin since low carbohydrate levels indicate lower insulin levels. A high diet of starch resembles putting petroleum on the insulin obstruction fire. A more influential need for insulin is indicated by elevated sugar, and this aggravates insulin opposition. A ketogenic diet, by correlation, turns down insulin levels since fat is the least insulin-requiring macronutrient. In comparison, bringing the insulin levels down also helps with fat intake, provided that elevated insulin levels inhibit fat breakdown. The body will differentiate fat cells at the point that insulin levels decrease for several hours.

4. Hypertension control

It is estimated that 16 million people in the U.K. suffer from hypertension. Hypertension, for example, cardiovascular disease, stroke, and renal disease, is related to the scope of health disorders. Different studies have demonstrated that a ketogenic diet can reduce circulatory stress levels in overweight or type 2 diabetes people. It is also a part of metabolic imbalance.

5. Cholesterol levels

For the most part, ketogenic diets bring in reductions in cholesterol levels. LDL cholesterol levels are usually reduced, and HDL cholesterol levels increase, which is healthy. The amount of absolute cholesterol to HDL is possibly the most substantiated proportion of safe cholesterol. It can be effectively detected by taking the full cholesterol result and partitioning it by your HDLS result. It indicates good cholesterol, on the off chance that the amount you get is 3.5 or lower. Study findings suggest that ketogenic diets are normally possible to increase this proportion of good cholesterol.

After starting a ketogenic, a few individuals can display an expansion in LDL and all-out cholesterol. It is generally taken as a bad indicator, but this does not speak of compounding in heart health if the absolute cholesterol to HDL ratio is appropriate.

Cholesterol is a confounding topic, and if your cholesterol levels essentially shift on a ketogenic diet, your PCP is the optimization technique of exhortation. More simple mental results. Other typically announced advantages of eating a ketogenic diet are emotional insight, an increased capacity to center, and superior memory. Expanding the admission of omega-3 healthy fats, such as those present in slick fish such as salmon, fish, and mackerel, will boost the state of mind and the ability to read. It is because omega-3 extends an unsaturated fat called DHAS, which makes up 15 to 30 percent of the cerebrum of females. The discovery of beta-hydroxybutyrate, a type of Ketone, allows for long-term memory work to be facilitated.

6. Satiety

The effects of ketogenic diets impact malnutrition. As the body responds to being in a ketosis state, it becomes acclimatized to obtain vitality from muscle to fat ratio differentiation, which will alleviate appetite and desires.

They are possible at:

- **Reducing desires**
- **Reducing inclination for sugary nourishments**
- **Helping you feel full for more**

Weight loss will also reduce leptin levels attributable to a ketogenic diet, which will increase the affectability of leptin and thus gain satiety.

1.4. Keto Shopping List

A keto diet meal schedule for women above 5o+ years and a menu that will transform the body. Generally speaking, the keto diet is low in carbohydrates, high in fat and moderate in protein. While adopting a ketogenic diet, carbs are routinely reduced to under 50 grams every day, but stricter and looser adaptations of the diet exist.

• Proteins can symbolize about 20 percent of strength requirements, whereas carbohydrates are usually restricted to 5 percent.

• The body retains its fat for the body to use as energy production.

Most of the cut carbs should be supplanted by fats and convey about 75% of your all-out caloric intake.

The body processes ketones while it is in ketosis, particles released from cholesterol in the blood glucose is low, as yet another source of energy.

Because fat is always kept a strategic distance from its unhealthy content, research demonstrates that the keto diet is essentially better than low-fat diets to advance weight reduction.

In contrast, keto diets minimize desire and improve
satiation, which is especially useful when getting in shape.

Fatty cuts of **PROTEIN**: *Keto Diet Shopping list*

NUTS AND SEEDS:
1. MACADAMIA NUTS+BUTTER
2. BRAZIL NUTS+BUTTER
3. PECANS+BUTTER
4. WALNUTS
5. PUMPKIN SEEDS
6. ALMONDS +BUTTER

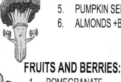

1. GROUND BEEF - RIBEYE STEAK
2. PORK BELLY ROAST +BACON
3. BEEF OR PORK SAUSAGE
4. WILD CAUGHT SALMON
5. SARDINES OR TUNA
6. CHICKEN THIGHS OR LEGS
7. TURKEY LEGS
8. DEER STEAKS
9. EGGS
10. DUCK EGGS
11.

Green Leafy **VEGGIES**:
1. BROCCOLI
2. CAULIFLOWER
3. GREEN BEANS
4. BRUSSEL SPROUTS
5. KALE
6. SPINACH
7. CHARD
8. CABBAGE
9. BOK CHOY
10. CELERY
11. ARUGULA
12. ASPARAGUS
13. ZUCCHINI
14. YELLOW SQUASH
15. MUSHROOMS
16. OLIVES
17. ARTICHOKE
18. CUCUMBERS
19. ONIONS
20. GARLIC
21. OKRA

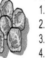

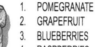

FATS:
1. BUTTER
2. OLIVE OIL
3. COCONUT OIL
4. COCONUT BUTTER
5. MCT OIL
6. AVOCADO
7. GHEE
8. BACON GREASE
9. AVOCADO OIL

FRUITS AND BERRIES:
1. POMEGRANATE
2. GRAPEFRUIT
3. BLUEBERRIES
4. RASPBERRIES
5. LEMON
6. LIME
7. AVOCADO

MUST HAVE MISCELLANEOUS:
1. ALMOND+COCONUT FLOUR
2. COCONUT BUTTER
3. 85% DARK CHOCOLATE
4. PORK RINDS
5. COCONUT CREAM
6. COCONUT FLAKES

1.5. Keto-Friendly Foods to Eat

Meals and bites should be based on the accompanying nourishment when following a ketogenic diet:

Eggs: pastured eggs are the best choice for all-natural eggs.

Meat: hamburger grass- nourished, venison, pork, organ meat, and buffalo.

Full-fat dairy: yogurt, cream and margarine.

Full-fat Cheddar: Cheddar, mozzarella, brie, cheddar goat and cheddar cream.

Nuts and seeds: almonds, pecans, macadamia nuts, peanuts, pumpkin seeds, and flaxseeds.

Poultry: turkey and chicken.

Fatty fish: Wild-got salmon, herring, and mackerel

Nut margarine: Natural nut, almond, and cashew spreads.

Vegetables that are not boring: greens, broccoli, onions, mushrooms, and peppers.

Condiments: salt, pepper, lemon juice, vinegar, flavors and crisp herbs.

Fats: coconut oil, olive oil, coconut margarine, avocado oil, and sesame oil.

Avocados: it is possible to add whole avocados to practically any feast or bite.

1.6. Nourishments to avoid

Although adopting a keto diet, keep away from carbohydrate-rich nutrients.

It is important to restrict the accompanying nourishments:

- **Sweetened beverages:** beer, juice, better teas, and drinks for sports.
- **Pasta:** noodles and spaghetti.
- **Grains and vegetable articles:** maize, rice, peas, oats for breakfast
- **Starchy vegetables:** Butternut squash, Potatoes, beans, sweet potatoes, pumpkin and peas.
- **Beans and vegetables:** chickpeas, black beans, kidney beans and lentils.
- **Fruit:** citrus, apples, pineapple and bananas.
- **Sauces containing high-carbohydrates:** BBQ' sauce, a sugar dressing with mixed greens, and dipping's.
- **Hot and bread items:** white bread, whole wheat bread, wafers, cookies, doughnuts, rolls, etc.
- **Sweets and sweet foods:** honey, ice milk, candy, chocolate syrup, agave syrup, coconut sugar.
- **Blended refreshments:** Sugar-blended cocktails and beer.

About the assumption that carbs should be small, low-glycemic organic goods, for example, when a keto-macronutrient is served, spread, berries may be satisfied with restricted quantities. Be sure to choose safe sources of protein and eliminate prepared sources of food and bad fats.

It is worth keeping the accompanying stuff away from:

1. Diet nutrients: Foods containing counterfeit hues, contaminants and carbohydrates, such as aspartame and sugar alcohols.

2. Unhealthy fats: Such as corn and canola oil, include shortening, margarine, and cooking oils.

3. Processed foods: Fast foods, bundled food sources, and frozen meats, such as wieners and meats for lunch.

1.8. One week Keto Diet Plan

(Day 1): Monday

Breakfast: Eggs fried in seasoned butter served over vegetables.

Lunch: A burger of grass-bolstered with avocado, mushrooms, and cheddar on a tray of vegetables.

Dinner: Pork chops and French beans sautéed in vegetable oil.

(Day 2): Tuesday

Breakfast: Omelet of mushroom.

Lunch: Salmon, blended vegetables, tomato, and celery on greens.

Dinner: Roast chicken and sautéed cauliflower.

(Day 3): Wednesday

Breakfast: Cheddar cheese, eggs, and bell peppers.

Lunch: Blended veggies with hard-bubbled eggs, avocado, turkey, and cheddar.

Dinner: Fried salmon sautéed in coconut oil.

(Day 4): Thursday

Breakfast: Granola with bested full-fat yogurt.

Lunch: Steak bowl of cheddar, cauliflower rice, basil, avocado, as well as salsa.

Dinner: Bison steak and mushy cauliflower.

(Day 5): Friday

Breakfast: Pontoons of Avocado egg (baked).

Lunch: Chicken served with Caesar salad.

Dinner: Pork, with veggies.

(Day 6): Saturday

Breakfast: Avocado and cheddar with cauliflower.

Lunch: Bunless burgers of salmon.

Dinner: Parmesan cheddar with noodles topped with meatballs.

(Day 7): Sunday

Breakfast: Almond Milk, pecans and Chia pudding.

Lunch: Cobb salad made of vegetables, hard-boiled eggs, mango, cheddar, and turkey.

Dinner: Curry chicken.

Chapter 2: Health Concerns for Women Over 50+

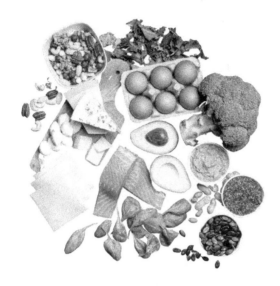

This chapter will give you a detailed view of the health concerns for women over 50.

2.1. Menopause

Healthy maturation includes large propensities such as eating healthy, avoiding regular prescription mistakes, monitoring health conditions, receiving suggested screenings, or being dynamic. Getting more seasoned involves change, both negative and positive, but you can admire maturing on the off chance of understanding your body's new things and finding a way to maintain your health. As you age, a wide range of things happens to your body. Unexpectedly, your skin, bones, and even cerebrum may start to carry on. Try not to let the advances that accompany adulthood get you off guard.

Here's a segment of the normal ones:

1. The Bones: In mature age, bones may become slender and progressively weaker, especially in women, leading to the delicate bone disease known as osteoporosis once in a while. Diminishing bones and decreasing bone mass can put you at risk for falls that can occur in broken bones without much of a stretch result. Make sure you talk to your doctor about what you can do to prevent falls and osteoporosis.

2. The Heart: While a healthy diet and normal exercise can keep your heart healthy, it may turn out to be somewhat amplified, lowering your pulse and thickening the heart dividers.

3. The Sensory system and Mind: It can trigger changes in your reflexes and even your skills by becoming more seasoned. While dementia is certainly not an ordinary outcome of mature age, individuals must encounter some slight memory loss as they become more stated. The formation of plaques and tangles, abnormalities that could ultimately lead to dementia, can harm cells in the cerebrum and nerves.

4. The Stomach: A structure associated with your stomach. As you age, it turns out that your stomach-related is all the more firm and inflexible and does not contract as often. For example, stomach torment, obstruction, and feelings of nausea can prompt problems with this change; a superior diet can help.

5. The Abilities: You can see that your hearing and vision is not as good as it ever was. Maybe you'll start losing your sense of taste. Flavors might not appear as unique to you. Your odor and expertise in touch can also weaken. In order to respond, the body requires more time and needs more to revitalize it.

6. The Teeth: Throughout the years, the intense veneer protecting your teeth from rot will begin to erode, making you exposed to pits. Likewise, gum injury is a problem for more developed adults. Your teeth and gums will guarantee great dental cleanliness. Dry mouth, which is a common symptom of seniors' multiple drugs, can also be a concern.

7. The Skin: Your skin loses its versatility at a mature age and can tend to droop and wrinkle. Nonetheless, the more you covered your skin when you were younger from sun exposure and smoke, the healthier your skin would look as you get more mature. Start securing your skin right now to prevent more injury, much like skin malignancy.

8. The Sexual Conviviality: When the monthly period ends following menopause, many women undergo physical changes such as vaginal oil loss. Men can endure erectile brokenness. Fortunately, it is possible to handle the two problems successfully.

A normal part of maturing is a series of substantial improvements, but they don't need to back you up. Furthermore, you should do a lot to protect your body and keep it as stable as you would imagine, given the circumstances.

2.2. Keys to Aging Well

Although good maturation must preserve your physical fitness, it is also vital to appreciate the maturity and growth you acquire with propelling years. Its fine to rehearse healthy propensities for an extraordinary period, but it's never beyond the point of no return to gain the benefits of taking great account of yourself, even as you get more developed.

Here are some healthy maturing tips at every point of life that are a word of wisdom:

- Keep dynamic physically with a normal workout.

- With loved ones and inside your locale, remain socially diverse.

- Eat a balanced, well-adjusted diet, dumping low-quality food to intake low-fat, fiber-rich, and low-cholesterol.

- Do not forget yourself: daily enrollment at this stage with your primary care provider, dental surgeon, and optometrist is becoming increasingly relevant.

- Taking all medications as the primary care provider coordinates.

- Limit the consumption of liquor and break off smoke.

- Receive the rest your body wants.

Finally, it is necessary to deal with your physical self for a long time, but it is vital that you still have an eye on your passionate health. Receive and enjoy the rewards of your long life every single day. It is the perfect chance to enjoy better health and pleasure.

1. Eat a healthy diet

For more developed development, excellent nourishment and sanitation are especially critical. You need to regularly ensure that you eat a balanced, tailored diet. To help you decide on astute diet options and practice healthy nutrition, follow these guidelines.

2. Stay away from common medication mistakes

Drugs can cure health conditions and allow you to continue to lead a long, stable life. Drugs may also cause real health problems at the stage that they are misused. To help you decide on keen decisions about the remedy and over-the-counter medications you take, use these assets.

3. Oversee health conditions

Working with your healthcare provider to monitor health issues such as diabetes, osteoporosis, and hypertension is important. To treat these regular health problems, you need to get familiar with the medications and gadgets used.

4. Get screened

Health scans are an effective means of helping to perceive health conditions - even before any signs or side effects are given. Tell the healthcare provider what direct health scans are for you to determine how much you can be screened.

5. Be active

Exercise, as well as physical action, can help you to remain solid and fit. You just don't have to go to an exercise center. Converse about proper ways that you really can be dynamic with your healthcare professional. Look at the assets of the FDA and our accomplices in the administration.

2.3. Skin Sagging

There are also ways to prevent age from sagging, which are:

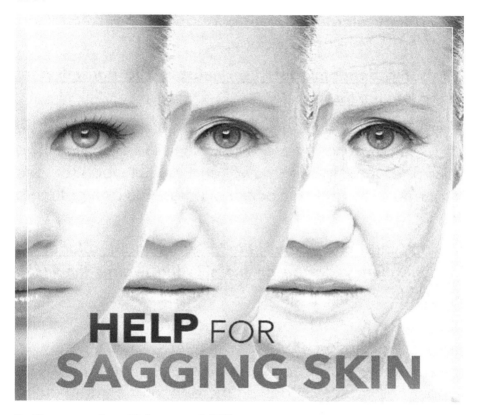

1. Unassuming Fixing and Lifting

These systems are called non-obtrusive methodologies of non-intrusive skin fixing on the basis that they leave your skin unblemished. A while later, you won't have a cut injury, a cut, or crude skin. You may see and grow some impermanent redness, but that is usually the main sign that you have a technique.

It is what you can expect from a skin-fixing method that is non-intrusive:

- **Results:** seem to come step by step, so they seem normal to be
- **Downtime:** zero to little
- **Colorblind:** secure for people with all skin hues
- **Body-wide use:** you can patch the skin almost anywhere on your body.

<u>Ultrasonic dermatologists use ultrasound to transmit heat deep into the tissue.</u>

Key concern: warming will induce more collagen to be created by your body. Many individuals see the unobtrusive raising and fixing within two and a half years of one procedure. By getting additional drugs, you can get more benefits.

<u>During this procedure, the dermatologist places a radiofrequency device on the skin that warms the tissue beneath.</u>

Key concern: Most people get one treatment and instantly feel an obsession. Your body needs some money to manufacture collagen, so you'll see the best effects in about half a year. By getting more than one treatment, a few persons benefit.

<u>Some lasers will send heat deeply through the skin without injuring the skin's top layer by laser therapy. These lasers are used to repair skin everywhere and can be especially effective for fixing free skin on the tummy and upper arms.</u>

Primary concern: to get outcomes, you may need 3 to 5 drugs, which occur step by step somewhere in the region of 2 and a half years after the last procedure.

2. Most fixing and lifting without medical procedure

While these methodologies will deliver you increasingly measurable results, considering all, they will not give you the aftereffects of an operation such as a facelift, eyelid surgical treatment, or neck lift, insignificantly pleasing to the eye skin fixing techniques. Negligibly obtrusive skin fixing requires less personal time than surgical treatment, however. It also conveys less chance of reactions.

3. How to look younger than your age without Botox, lasers and surgery, plus natural remedies for skin sagging

It is possible to become more experienced in this lifetime. However, you don't need to look at your age on the off chance you'd like not to. Truth be told, if you have been wondering how you would look as youthful as you feel, we will be eager to bet that you feel a lot more youthful than the amount you call your "age!"

2.4. Weight loss

Quality preparation builds the quality of your muscles and improves your versatility.

Even though cardio is very important for lung health and the heart, getting more fit and keeping it off is anything but an incredible technique.

The weight will return quickly at the point when you quit doing a lot of cardio. An unquestionable requirement has cardio as a component of your general wellness routine; be that as it may, when you start going to the exercise centre, quality preparation should be the primary factor. Quality preparation increases your muscle's quality, but this will enhance your portability and the main thing known to build bone thickness (alongside appropriate supplements).

Weight-bearing exercises help build and maintain bulk and build bone quality and reduce the risk of osteoporosis. Many people over [the age of] 50 will stop regularly practicing due to torment in their joints or back or damage, but do not surrender. In any case, understand that because of age-related illness, hormone changes, and even social variables such as a busy life, it may seem more enthusiastic to pick up muscle as you age. As he would like to think that to build durable muscles, cardio will consume off fat and pick substantial weights with few representatives or lighter weights. Similarly, for generally speaking health and quality, remember exercise and diet are linked to the hip, likewise, as the trick of the year. ! Locate a professional who can help you get back into the groove and expect to get 2 hrs. Thirty minutes of physical movement in any case [in] seven days to help to maintain your bulk and weight.

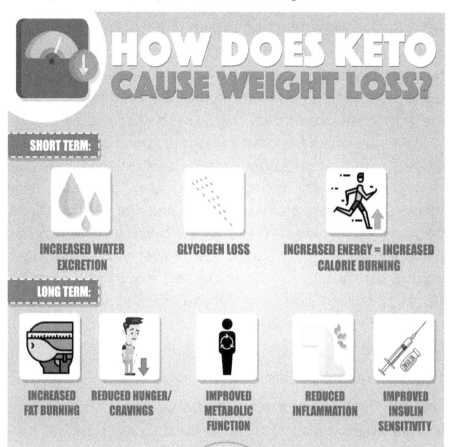

1. Try not to skip meals.

Testosterone and Estrogen decline gradually after some time, which also prompts fat collection because the body does not prepare sugar. We alternatively keep losing more bulk as we get older; this will cause our bodies' metabolic needs to lessen. Be that as it may, meal skipping can make you lack significant key medications required as we age, for example, by before large protein and calories. Tracking your energy levels throughout the day and obtaining sufficient calories/protein would also help you feel better on the scale, explaining how you will be burning more calories but less inefficiently. We also lose more bulk as we age, causing our metabolic rate to decrease. Be that as it may, skipping meals can make you lack important key supplements required as we age, for example, by an aging, metabolic rate.

2. Ensure you are getting enough rest.

"Perhaps the highest argument of over 50 years is a lack of rest," Amselem notes. Basically, rest may interfere with an important medical procedure, causing metabolic breakage in the system, in which the body turns weakness into hunger, urging you to eat. I plan to rest for seven to eight hours and, if necessary, take low rest. Rest is vital to a healthy weight because two hormones, leptin, and Ghrelin are released during rest, and they conclude a significant job in eating guidelines.

3. Relinquish old "rules" about weight loss and develop an outlook on health.

For the two women and men, age impacts weight loss, and that is on the basis that digestion backs off, hormone levels decay, in addition to there is a loss of bulk," "Nevertheless, that does not imply that mission is inconceivable to get more fit over age 50. Everybody else has to take a half hour's exercise, but there are two big reasons why it can't be done: you eat too much, or you are not active enough. The wellness movement encourages people to be aware of their own health, body and well-being. Being over 50 years old is not the end of the world. In fact, there is still a chance for us to live the rest of our lives as retirees. It is important to eat well, exercise, not smoke, and limit alcohol consumption in our lives. Our bodies are naturally aging, but we do not yet have to quit. Instead of falling prey to craze diets, make ongoing acclimatization to advance adjusted eating, and help yourself remember the benefits of exercise for your heart, stomach-related tract, and psychological well-being, despite the executives' weight.

2.5. Factors Influencing Fuel Utilization

The amount of each element in one's blood plasma determines the combination of fuels in the body. According to the researchers, the main element that determines how much of each nutrient is absorbed is the quantity of each nutrient eaten first by the body. The second considerations to take into account when assessing one's health is the amounts of hormones like insulin and glucagon, which must be in balance with one's diet. The third is the body's physical accumulation (cellular) of any nutrient, such as fat, muscle, and liver glycogen. Finally, the quantities of regulatory enzymes for glucose & fat breakdown beyond our influence, but changes in diet and exercise decide each gasoline's overall usage. Surely, both of these considerations will be discussed more extensively below.

1. Quantity of nutrients consumed

Humans will obtain four calories from sources in their surroundings: carbon, hydrogen, nitrogen, and oxygen. When it comes to the body demanding and using a given energy supply, it prefers to choose the nearest one to it due to the quantity and concentration in the bloodstream. The body can improve its use of glucose or decrease its use of glucose directly due to the amount of carbohydrate intake being ingested. It is an effort by the liver to control glycogen (sugar) levels in the body. If carbohydrate (carb) intake goes up, the use of carbohydrate-containing goods will go up, in exchange. Proteins are slightly harder to control. As protein consumption goes up, our bodies increase their development and oxidation of proteins as well. The food source for our body is protein. If it is in short supply, our body will consume less of it. This is an attempt to keep body protein cellular levels stable at 24-hour intervals. Since dietary fat does not lift the amount of fat the body needs, it cannot dramatically change how much fuel the body gets from that fat. Rather than measuring insulin directly, it is important to measure insulin indirectly, so it does not drift.

The blood alcohol content can decrease the body's energy reserves with those calories of fat. This will almost entirely impair the body's usage of fat for food. As most people know, carbohydrate intake will influence the amount of fat the body uses as a fuel supply. High carb diets increase the body's use of fat for food and the insulin threshold and amount. Therefore, the highest fat oxidation rates occur when there are low levels of carbohydrates in the body. Another clarification of this can be found in chapter 18, where it is clarified that the amount of glycogen regulates how much fat is used by the muscles. When a human eats less energy and carbohydrates, the body can subsequently take up fat calories for food instead of carbohydrates.

2. Hormone levels

Factors like food, exercise, medications and hormones all play a part in how we use our bodies' fuel. The hormone known as insulin is of high interest to many physicians because it plays a significant role in a wide range of activities, including the bodies functioning. A glance at the hormones involved in fuel consumption is included in the following passage.

Insulin is a peptide (as in the "peptide" in "peptides" that are essential in digestion) that the pancreas releases in response to changes in blood glucose. As blood glucose goes up, insulin levels also rise, and the body will use this extra glucose to kind of store it as glycogen in the muscles or in the liver. Glucose and extra glucose will be forced into fat cells for preservation (as alpha-glycerophosphate). Protein synthesis is enhanced, and as a result, amino acids (the building blocks of proteins) are transferred out of the blood via muscle cells and are then placed together to make bigger proteins. Fat synthesis or "lipogenesis" (making fat) and fat accumulation are also induced. In effect, it's hard for insulin to be released from fat cells due to even tiny levels of it. The main objective of insulin is regulating blood glucose in a very small range of around 80 to 120 milligrams per decilitre. When blood glucose levels rise outside of the normal range, insulin is released to get the glucose levels back into a normal range. The greatest rise in blood glucose levels (and the greatest increase in insulin) happens when humans eat carbohydrates in the diet. Due to amino acids that can be converted to glycogen, the breakdown of proteins can cause an increase the amount of insulin released. FFA can induce insulin release and produce ketone bodies found at concentrations that are far smaller than those produced by carbohydrates or proteins.

When your glucose level decreases, as it does with exercise and from eating less carbohydrate, your insulin levels decrease as well. During cycles with low insulin and higher hormones, the body's storage fuels can burst, leading to a breakdown of stored fuels. After accumulation within the body, triglycerides are broken down into fatty acids and glycerol and released into the bloodstream. Specific proteins might be broken down into individual amino acids and used as sources of sources glucose. Glycogen is a material contained in the liver that is broken when insulin is absent. Failure to produce insulin suggests a pathological state. Type me, diabetes (or Insulin Dependent Diabetes Mellitus, IDDM). In a group of patients with Type I diabetes (1), these patients have a deficiency in the pancreas, causing them to be entire without insulin. I already told you that to practical control glucose levels, people with diabetes have to inject themselves with insulin. This is relevant in the next chapter since the difference between diabetic ketoacidosis and dietary mediated ketosis is made in the chapter after this. Glucagon is essentially known as insulin's mirror hormone in the body and has nearly opposite effects. The enzyme insulin is also a peptide hormone made by the pancreas, which is released from the cells of the body, and its primary function as well is to sustain stable glucose levels. However, once blood glucose goes down below average, glucagon increases blood glucose on its own. The precursors are expelled from the cells into the bloodstream.

Glucagon's key function is in the liver, where it signals the degradation of liver glycogen and the resulting release into the bloodstream. The release of glucagon is modulated by what we eat, the sort of workout, and the presence of a meal that activates the development of glucagon in the body (24). High amounts of insulin suppress the pancreas from releasing the hormone glucagon. Normally, glucagon's actions are restricted to the liver; by comparison, its function in these other tissues is yet to be detected (i.e., fat and muscle cells). On the other hand, when insulin levels are very low, such as when glucose restriction and activity occur, glucagon plays a minor role in fat mobilization, as well as the degradation of muscle glycogen. Glucagon's primary function is to regulate blood glucose under conditions of low blood sugar. But it also plays a crucial role in ketone body development in the liver, which we will address in-depth in the next chapter. Below are the definitions of two contrasting hormones. It should be obvious from reading the sentences that they have opposite effects on one another. Whereas insulin is a key storage hormone that allows for the retention of accumulated glucose, potassium, albumin and fat in the body, glucagon serves the same role by allowing for the utilization of stored fat in an organism.

Insulin and glucagon are central to the determination to be anabolic or catabolic. However, their presence in the body is not alone enough for muscle development. Other hormones are involved as well. They will briefly be discussed below. Growth hormone, which is a peptide hormone, elicits various effects on the body, such as its effects on blood flow and muscle tissue growth. The hormone to hold appetite at bay, Ghrelin, is released in response to several stressors. Most notably, exercise, a reduction in blood glucose, and carbohydrate restriction or fasting can both induce Ghrelin production. As its name suggests (GH), GH is a growth-promoting hormone, which enhances protein production (protein synthesis) in the body and liver. Glucose, glycogen, and triglycerides also are mobilized from fat cells for nutrition.

Adrenaline and noradrenaline (also called epinephrine and norepinephrine) are members of a special family of hormones called 'fight or flight' hormones. They tend to be released in response to discomfort, such as running, fasting, or consuming cold foods. Epinephrine is a drug that is emitted from the adrenal medulla, passing across the bloodstream to the brain to exert its effects on several tissues of the body. The impacts of the catecholamine's on the different tissues of the body are very involved and maybe the subject of a research paper. The primary function of catecholamine metabolites affecting the ketogenic diet was to increase fatty acids excretion in the urine and increase fatty acids in the blood. When it's hard for someone to change their ways, it's because their insulin levels aren't where they should be. The only hormone that actually affects fat mobilization is insulin. Like the

Catecholamine's, insulin and insulin mimics have a corresponding effect on fat mobilization.

3. Liver glycogen

The liver is one of the most metabolically active organs in the whole human body. Although everything we consume is not digested immediately by the stomach, this is part of the whole digestion process. Like the body, the degree to which the liver retains glycogen is the dominating influence to the extent to which the body will retain or break down nutrients. It is typically (hesitation) because there is a higher body fat level associated with elevated liver glycogen levels. The liver is analogous to a short term stead storehouse and glycogen source regulating blood glucose in our body. After the liver releases more glucose into the blood, more glucagon is released, which activates the breaking down of liver glycogen to glucose, to be introduced into the bloodstream. When the liver has glycogen stocks completely, blood glucose levels are retained, and the body enters the anabolic state, meaning the incoming glucose, amino acids, and free fatty acids are all processed as these three molecules, respectively. This is often referred to as 'the fed establishment.' Red blood cells can't hold as much oxygen as they did when filled with massive amounts of glycogen, so they release it when they're no longer needed and transform into the liver. The body cuts edible protein into amino acids, which are then placed into the formation of amino acids, and finally, will produce for you fats and sugars. This is often referred to as the 'fasted' condition.

4. Enzyme levels

Precise control of fuel consumption in the body is done through the action of enzymes. Ultimately, enzyme levels are calculated by the carbohydrates that are being consumed in the diet and the hormone levels which are caused by it. On the other hand, where there is a surplus of carbohydrates in one's diet, this form of dietary shift stimulates insulin's influence on the cells' ability to utilize glucose and prevent fatty stores' degradation. Thus, if there is a decrease in insulin levels, the enzymes are blocked, which results in a drop in the enzymes involved in glucose usage and in fats breakdown. A long term adjustment to a high carbohydrate / low carbohydrate diet may induce longer-term modifications in the enzymes involved in fats and carbohydrates, resulting in long term changes in the core. If you limit carbohydrate consumption for many weeks, this will deplete enzymes' liver and muscle and transfer them to be brought upon the liver and muscle that concerns fat burning. The result of disrupting the balance of dietary components is an inability to use carbs for fuel for some time after food is reintroduced to the diet.

Chapter 3: Keto with Intermittent Fasting

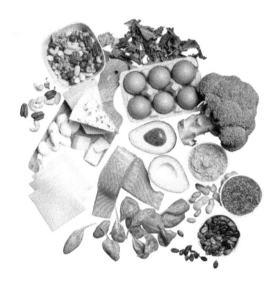

This chapter will give you a detailed view to the Keto with intermittent fasting.

Intermittent fasting, in a more condensed definition, allows people to miss a meal daily. The popular forms of intermittent fasting include the one day fast, a 24 hour fast or a 5:2 fast, where people eat very little food for a predetermined number of days, then consume lots of food (ADF). The intermittent fasting function of IF breaks the subjects fasting routine every other day. Unlike crash diets that frequently produce rapid results but can be hard to sustain for the long run, both intermittent fasting and keto Diet focus on the real root systems of how the body absorbs food and how you make your dietary decisions for each day. Intermittent eating and Keto diets should be practiced as dietary modification. They are long-term options for a better, happier you.

It is where the biggest distinction lies among IF and Interval feeding (TRF). The TRF is the fast of restricting the feeding time to between 4-10 hours during the day and missing the fasting time the rest of the time. All or most people who observe intermittent fasting do so regularly.

3.1. What Is Ketosis?

From the outside looking in, carbs appear to be a simple and fast means of bringing nutrients right through the day. Think of all those grab-and-go and protein-filled snacks that we equate with breakfast—granola bars, fruit-filled muffins, smoothies. We start our mornings by eating many carbs, and then later on in the day, they add more carbs. Just because a given technology works does not make it the most effective way. To keep us safe, the tissues and cells that produce our bodies require energy to fulfil their daily functions. There are two main sources of strength in the foods we consume, but the first source is non-animal, and the second source is animal. One source of energy is the carbohydrate, which transforms into glucose. At this time, this is the process that most people go through. These cars have an alternative fuel, however, and a shocking one: fat. No, the very thing any doctor has recommended you to reduce your lifelong lifespan may be the weapon you need to jump-start your metabolism. During this process, tiny organic molecules, called Ketone, are emitted from our body, signalling that the food we eat is being broken down. Ketones are actual nutrients that help run much of our body's cells, including muscles. You've undoubtedly heard the term "Metabolism" repeated in one's life, but do you understand what it means exactly as a fast-acting chemical process? In short, this is alkaline, causing effective cellular functioning, which can be present in any type of living thing. Considering that humans are extremely difficult in many ways, our bodies generally process simpler things like food and exercise. Our bodies are actively struggling to do their jobs. And whether we are either asleep or not, our cells are actively constructing and restoring. The robots ought to remove the energetic particles from inside our bodies.

Around the same time, glucose, which is what carbohydrates are broken down into after we ingest them, is a critical component in the process of bringing sugar into the body. We are now concentrating our diet on carbs as the main source of calories for our body. Without mentioning the fructose we eat as well as the recommended daily servings of fruit, starchy veggies, and starchy vegetables, as well as plant-based sources of protein, there is no shortage of glucose in our bodies. The problem with this type of energy use is that this results in us buying into the recycling-focused consumerism that is a by-product of the half-baked technologies. Our bodies get hammered by the number of calories we eat every day. Some people are eating more than they need, and that can contribute to obesity.

Most people cannot reach ketosis quickly, but you can reach it by exercising, eating less, and drinking a decent amount of water. As was seen through the data, our current "Food Pyramid," which instructs us to consume a high amount of carbohydrate-rich foods as energy sources, is turned upside down. A more effective formula for feeding your body has fats at the top, making up 60 to 80 percent of your diet; protein in the middle at 20 to 30 percent; and carbs (real glucose in disguise) way at the bottom, accounting for only 5 to 10 percent of your regular eating plan.

3.2. Paleo vs. Keto

Evolution has many opportunities to bring. We can use fire and energy to cook our food is evidence enough that change can be a positive thing about our lives. Anywhere between our trapper foraging lifestyle and the industrialized lifestyle we have today, there is a significant disconnect. Although our lifespans have improved, we're not winning from the longevity of those additional years because our health is being undermined. The tired, unclear sensation you are having might be not just because you need to get more sleep - it may be because you lack vitamin B12 in your diet. If we eat food as fuel for our bodies, it's fair to assume that what we eat has a big effect on our productivity. If you burn fuel in an engine designed to run on gasoline, there could be some very harmful consequences. Is it conceivable that our bodies have set up this insulin receptor cascade to only accept sugar, in a process comparable to our transition to providing fat as a rapid source of energy rather than a source of energy for our early ancestors? I know this sounds an awful lot like arguing for a Paleo diet, but although the ketogenic lifestyle seems similar, keto's basic concept is vastly different. Ketosis happens when you eat fewer calories and change the intake of protein and fat. There are many medicinal effects of ketosis, and the primary one is quick weight loss (fat, protein, carbohydrates, fiber, and fluids). Per calorie is made up of four distinct types of macronutrients. Many considerations go into the certain food decisions that a person makes, and it's crucial to consider one's emotions.

Fiber makes us regular, for instance, and it lets food flows into the digestive tract. What goes in has to come out, and for that process, fiber is necessary. Protein helps to heal tissue, generate enzymes and to create bones, muscles and skin. Liquids keep us hydrated; our cells, muscles, and organs do not operate correctly without them. The primary function of carbohydrates is to supply energy, but the body must turn them into glucose to do so, which has a ripple effect on the body's parts. Because of its link to insulin production through higher blood sugar levels, a carb intake is a balancing act for persons with diabetes. Good fats stimulate cell formation, protect our lungs, help keep us warm, and supply nutrition, but only in small amounts when carbs are ingested. I'm going to explain more about when and how this is happening soon.

3.3. Carbs vs. Net Carbs

In virtually any food supply, carbohydrates occur in some type. Total carbohydrate reduction is unlikely and unrealistic. To work, we want some carbohydrates. If we want to learn that certain foods that drop into the restricted group on a keto diet become better options than others, it's important to understand this.

In the caloric breakdown of a meal, fiber counts as a carb. It is interesting to remember is that our blood sugar is not greatly impaired by fiber, a positive thing because it is an integral macronutrient that allows us better digest food. You're left with what's considered net carbs after subtracting the sum of fiber from the number of carbs in the caloric tally of an element or finished recipe. Think of your pay check before (gross) taxes and after (net). A bad comparison, maybe, because no one wants to pay taxes, but an efficient one to try to explain and track carbs versus net carbs. You place a certain amount of carbohydrates in your bloodstream, but any of them does not influence your blood sugar content.

It doesn't mean that with whole-grain pasta, you may go mad. Although it's a better alternative than flour of white-coloured pasta, you can limit your net carbs to 20 - 30 grams per day total. To place that in context, approximately 35 g of carbohydrates and just 7 grams of total fiber are found in two ounces of undercooked whole-grain pasta. Pasta and bread are undoubtedly the two key things people would ask you if you miss them.

3.4. When does ketosis kick in?

Most individuals go through ketosis within a few days. People who are different will take a week to adapt. Factors that cause ketosis include existing body mass, diet, and exercise levels. Ketosis is a moderate state of ketosis since ketone levels would be low for a longer time. One can calculate ketone levels in a structured way, but you can note certain biological reactions that indicate you are in ketosis. There are not as serious or drastic symptoms, and benefits can outweigh risks in this phase-in time, so it is good to be familiar with symptoms in case they arise.

Starvation vs. Fasting

Make a deliberate decision to fast. The biggest differentiator between going on a fast and feeding intermittently is that it is your choice to continue fasting. The amount of time you want to fast and the reason for fasting are not imposed upon you by the hospital, whether it is for religious practices, weight loss, or a prolonged detox cycle. Most fasting is performed at will. When fasting, proper feeding has clear implications on the overall way of our well-being. A series of situations can bring about starvation out of the hands of the people suffering from those conditions. Starvation, hunger, and war are but a couple of these conditions to be caused by a devastated economy. Starvation is starvation due to lack of the proper nutrients that can lead to organ failure and ultimately death. No one wants to live without calories.

When I knew that avoiding smoking would help my health, I immediately wondered, "Why do I continue to smoke?"

And once I learn about the motivations for doing this, it is much easier to see them. I have also been concerned about the early days of fasting. Before I knew that there is a distinction between fasting and starvation and that it is safe, my first response to the thought of not eating and starving was still, "Why would anyone choose to kill themselves with starving?." As for this article's intent, someone who fasts is just opting not to eat for a predetermined amount of time. Even nonviolent vigils that are meant to oppose using a certain form of killing feed larger and larger gatherings.

Would your hunger vanish before the fast?

So that's a brilliant query; let's try a couple more angles. The fact is, we all eat a full meal once a day. It is a normal tradition that we eat our last meal a few hours before going to sleep, and all but breastfeeding new-borns do not eat the moment they wake up. And if you devote just a limit of six hours a night to sleep, you are likely to be fasting ten hours a day anyway. Now, let's begin to incorporate the concept in periodic to the formula. Anything that is "intermittent" implies something that is not constant. When adding it to the concept of fasting, it means you're lengthening the time that you don't eat between meals (the term "breakfast" means only that, breaking the fast).

From fasting once a day, we have an established "mind over matter" power. What will be a major concern, though, would be mind over mind. We will come back to the issue of how you feel after you stop feeding. The first week of fasting may change as you get used to the prolonged amount of time of your current intermittent fasting target. All of the fasting periods that I have given allow you time-wise to adapt to the Ketogenic Diet and this method adjusts your sleeping routine so that it suits them. It is conceivable (and likely) that your body will start to feel hungry about 10 a.m., around the moment it usually eats lunch. But, after one day, you can adapt, and after a couple of days, you should no longer have trouble feeding before noon.

To support you before making the shift you're playing with, observe what happens when you put back the first meal of the day by an extra thirty minutes per day for a week. This way, as you begin the schedule set out here, you'll need to change the timing of your final meal of the day just after you begin week two of the plan for the Meals from Noon to 6 p.m. No appointments are required.

3.5. Why Prefer Intermittent Fasting?

Now that you have learned that it is possible to fast without starving to death and that it is also a deliberate decision, you might think, why on earth you would ever choose to fast. Its ability to encourage weight loss is one of the key reasons that IF has taken the diet world by storm. Metabolism is one feature of the human body. Metabolism requires two basic reactions: catabolism and anabolism.

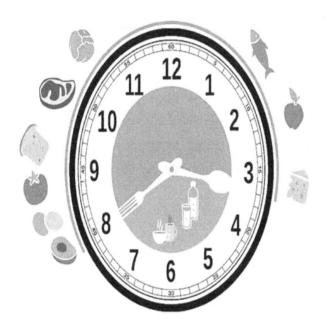

Catabolism is the portion of metabolism where our bodies break down food. Catabolism involves breaking down large compounds into smaller units. The body uses the energy from the food we consume to produce new cells, build muscles, and sustain organs. This term is often referred to as parallel or dual catabolism and anabolism. A diet routine that sees us eating most of the day means our bodies have less time to waste in the anabolic process of metabolism. It is hard to find out since they are related, but note that they occur at different rates. The most significant point is that a prolonged fasting time allows for optimum metabolic efficiency.

The improved mental acuity has an intrinsic influence of improving attention, focus, concentration and focus. According to various reports, fasting made you more alert and concentrated, not sleepy or light-headed. Many people point to nature and our desire to survive. We may not have had food preservation, but we lived day to day, regardless of how ample food supplies may have been.

Scientists agree that fasting often heightens neurogenesis, the growth and regeneration of nerve tissue in the brain. Both paths lead to the fact that fasting gives the body enough time to do routine maintenance. You extend the time you give your body to concentrate on cellular growth and tissue recovery by sleeping longer between your last meal and your first meal.

Are Fluids Allowed While Fasting?

The last important detail for intermittent fasting is that it speeds up the metabolism; unlike religious fasting, which also forbids food consumption during the fast period, an IF requires you to drink a certain liquid during the fast time. You are not consuming something that is caloric; therefore, this action breaks the fast. As we can glean from its strong weight loss record, a closer look through the prism of intermittent fasting can yield very promising outcomes. Bone broth (here) is the beneficiary of both the nutrients and vitamins and can refill the sodium amounts. Permission has been given to use coffee and tea without any sweeteners and ideally without any milk or cream. There are two separate schools of thinking about applying milk or soda to your coffee or tea. Provided it's just a high-fat addition, such as coconut oil or butter to make bulletproof coffee (here), many keto supporters believe it's a waste of time and not properly gain sufficient protein. Using MCT oil, it is assumed that people can obtain more energy and be happier moving on with their daily lives. Coffee and tea drinkers tend toward simple brews. It is perfect for you to choose whichever strategy you want, as long as you don't end up "alternating" between the two techniques. I often recommend drinking water, as staying hydrated is necessary for any healthier choice a person can make. Caffeine use can be very depleting, so be careful to control your water intake and keep yourself balanced.

3.6. The Power of Keto Combined & Intermittent Fasting

When you're in ketosis, the process breaks down fatty acids to create ketones for fuel is basically what the body does to keep things going when you're fasting. Fasting for a few days has a noticeable impact on a carb-based diet. After the initial step of burning carbohydrates for energy, your body transforms to burning fat for heat. You see where I'm going. If it takes 24 to 48 hrs. For the body to turn to fat for food, imagine the consequences of keto. Maintaining ketosis means your body has been trying to burn fat for fuel. Spending a long time in a fasting state means you burn fat. Intermittent starvation combined with keto results in more weight loss than other traditional diets. Extra fat-burning capabilities are due to the gap in time between the last and first meals. Ketosis is used in bodybuilding because it helps shed fat without losing muscle. It's healthy when it's the right weight, and muscle mass is good for fitness.

How does it work?

It is an incredible lifestyle adjustment to turn to the keto diet. Since it can help you consume less, it's better to ease into this program's fasting part. Despite the diet not being entirely fresh, yet has been around for a long time, people seem to respond rapidly to consuming mostly fat, so their body has been accustomed to burning fat for food, but be patient if either of the above occurs: headaches, exhaustion, light-headedness, dizziness, low blood sugars, nausea. A rise in appetite, cravings for carbohydrates, or weight gain. Often make sure you get certain nutrients: brain well-being, fat-burning, testosterone, and mood. Week 2 of the 4-Week schedule begins intermittent fasting, and it is not continued until the 2nd week. During the phase-in process, you'll want to find out what the meals and hours are about. Before integrating the intermittent-fasting portion of your diet, it is recommended that you stop eating your last meal more than six hours in advance. (6 p.m.) It will help you get into a fasting state and help you stop snacking. When you learn how to better nourish your body, you will learn how to reel in the pesky compulsion to feed, and you will be able to maintain a more controlled relationship with your psychological needs as well. When time goes by, cravings inevitably stop. We sometimes associate the craving for food with hunger, when actually the craving for food is due to a learned habit and hunger is a biochemical cue to refuel the body's energy stores.

3.7. Calories vs. Macronutrients

The focus on keto is on tracking the amount of fat, protein, and carbohydrates you eat. It's just a closer examination of every calorie ingested. To decide how many calories you can consume for weight management and weight loss, it is also important to have a baseline metabolic rate called BMR (another reason defining your goals is important). In both your general well-being and achieving and remaining in ketosis, all these macronutrients play a crucial function, but carbohydrates are the one that receives the most attention on keto since they result in glucose during digestion, which is the energy source you are attempting to guide your body away from utilizing. Any study indicates that the actual number of total carbs that one can eat a day on keto is 50 grams or less, resulting in 20 to 35 net carbs a day depending on the fiber content. The lower the net carbohydrates you can get down, the sooner your body goes into ketosis, and the better it's going to be to keep in it.

Bearing in mind that we target around 20 grams of net carbs a day, depending on how many calories you need to eat depending on your BMR, the fat and protein grams are factors. Depending on the exercise level, the recommended daily average for women ranges between 1,600 and 2,000 calories for weight maintenance (from passive to active). According to a daily diet, consuming 160 grams of fat + 70 grams of protein + 20 grams of carbohydrates represents 1,800 calories of intake, the optimal number for weight control for moderately active women in the USDA (walking 1.5 to 3 miles a day). You would like to reach for 130 grams of fat + 60 grams of protein + 20 grams of carbohydrates to jump-start weight loss if you have a sedentary lifestyle, described as having exercise from normal daily activities such as cleaning and walking short distances only (1500 calories).

3.8. The Physical Side Effects of Keto:

Unlike diet programs that merely reduce the weight loss foods you consume, keto goes further. In order to improve how the body turns what you consume into electricity, ketosis is about modifying the way you eat. The ketosis phase changes the equation from burning glucose (remember, carbs) to burning fat for fuel instead. When the body adapts to a different way of working, this comes with potential side effects. This is also why around week two, and not from the get-go, the 4-Week schedule here stages of intermittent fasting. It's important to give yourself time to change properly, both physically and mentally. Keto fever and keto breath are two physical alterations that you may encounter while transitioning to a keto diet.

1. Keto Flu

Often referred to as carb flu, keto flu can last anywhere from a few days to a few weeks. As the body weans itself from burning glucose for energy, metabolic changes occurring inside can result in increased feelings of lethargy, muscle soreness, irritability, light-headedness or brain fog, changes in bowel movements, nausea, stomach aches, and difficulty concentrating and focusing. It sounds bad, I know, and perhaps slightly familiar. Yes, these are all recurrent flu signs, hence the term. The good news is that when your body changes, this is a transient process, and it does not affect everybody. A deficiency of electrolytes (sodium, potassium, magnesium and calcium) and sugar removal from substantially reduced carbohydrate intake are reasons causing these symptoms. Expecting these future effects means that, should anything arise at all, you will be prepared to relieve them and reduce the duration of keto flu.

Sodium levels are specifically affected by the volume of heavily processed foods you eat. To explain, all we eat is a processed food; the word means "a series of steps taken to achieve a specific end." The act of processing food also involves cooking from scratch at home. However, these heavily processed foods appear to produce excessive amounts of secret salt in contrast to our present society, where ready-to-eat foods are available at any turn of the store (sodium is a preservative as well as a flavour modifier).

Other foods to concentrate on during your keto phase-in time are given below. They're a rich supply of minerals such as magnesium, potassium and calcium to keep the electrolytes in check.

- Potassium is important for hydration. It is present in Brussels sprouts, asparagus, salmon, tomatoes, avocados, and leafy greens.
- Seafood, Avocado, Spinach, Fish, and Vegetables that are high in magnesium can greatly assist with Cramps and Muscle Soreness.
- Calcium can promote bone health and aid in the absorption of nutrients.
- Including cheese, nuts, and seeds like almonds, broccoli, bok Choy, sardines, lettuce, sesame and chia seeds.

The other option that people evaluate to prevent the keto flu is to start eating less refined carbohydrates to lessen the chances of experiencing the keto flu. It can be as simple as making a few simple changes in what you eat, replacing the muffin with a hard-boiled or scrambled egg, replacing the bun with lettuce (often referred to as protein-style when ordering), or switching out spaghetti with zoodles. This way, when you dive into the plan here or here, it'll feel more like a gradual step of eating fewer carbohydrates than a sudden right turn in your diet.

2. Keto Breath

Let's dig into the crux of the matter first. Poor breath is basically a stench. But, it's a thing you can prepare yourself for when transitioning to the ketosis diet. There are two related hypotheses there might be a reason for this. When the body reaches ketosis (a state whereby it releases a lot of energy), which makes your fat a by-product of acid, more acetone is released by the body (yes, the same solvent found in nail polish remover and paint thinners). Any acetone is broken down in the bloodstream in a process called decarboxylation in order to get it out of the body into the urine and breathe in the acetone. It can cause that a person has foul-smelling breath.

When protein is also present in the keto breath, it adds a mildly gross sound. You must note that the macronutrient target is a high fat, mild protein, and low carb. People make the mistake that high fat is interchangeable with high protein. It is not a real assertion at all. The body's metabolism between fat and protein varies. Our bodies contain ammonia when breaking down protein, and all of the ammonia is normally released in our urine production. When you eat more protein or more than you should, the excess protein is not broken or digested and goes to your gut. With time, the extra protein will turn to ammonia and releasing by your breath.

3.9. The Fundamentals of Ketogenic Diet

The keto diet regimen involves eating moderately low carb, high sugar, and mild protein to train the body to accept fat as its basic food. Continuing the procedure, I would add a

Keto diet to my diet. Since the body may not have carbohydrate stores, it burns through its glycogen supplies rapidly. It is when the body appears to be in a state of emergency since it has run out of food. At this stage, the body goes into ketosis, and this is when you start using fat as the primary source of power. It typically occurs within three days of beginning the drug. Then, the body transforms the fat onto itself, usually taking over three months and a half to complete the transition. You are well accustomed to fat. So if you aren't feeding the body properly, that's why the body takes advantage of your own fat deposits (fasting).

The Keto Diet Advantage for Intermittent Fasting

Before entering intermittent fasting, keto advises four a month and a half to be on the keto diet. You're not going to be better off eating fat alone, so you're going to have less yearning. The keto diet in contemplates was all the more satisfying, and people encountered less yearning. In contrast, keto also showed its bulk storage ability and was best at maintaining digestion.

Sorts of Intermittent Fasting

This technique involves fasting two days a week and on some days actually eating 500 calories. You will have to observe a typical, healthy keto diet for the next five days. Because fasting days are allotted just 500 calories, you will need to spend high-protein and fat nutrients to keep you satisfied. Only made mindful that there is a non-fasting day in the middle of both.

1. Time-Restricted Eating

For the most part, because your fasting window involves the time you are dozing, this fasting approach has proven to be among the most popular. The swift 16/8 means that you are fast for sixteen hours and eat for eight hours. That might believe it is only allowed to eat from early afternoon until 8 p.m. and start quickly until the next day. The incredible thing about this technique is that it doesn't have to be 16/8; at the moment, you can do 14/10 and get equivalent incentives.

2. Interchange Day Fasting

Despite the 5:2 strategy and time restriction, this alternative allows you to be rapid every other day, normally limiting yourself from around 500 calories on fasting. The non-fasting days would actually be consumed normally. It can be an exhausting strategy that can make others hesitate when it is difficult to keep up with it.

3. 24 Hour Fast

I called, for short, "One Meal a Day" or OMAD, otherwise. This speed is sustained for an entire 24 hours and is usually done just a few days a week. Next, you'll need some inspiration to resume fasting to prop you up.

Keeping up the Motivation

It can be hard to stick to an eating and fasting regimen on the off chance that you are short on ideas, so how do you keep it up? The accompanying focus will help to concentrate on your general goals by presenting basic path reasons.

Chapter 4: Top 20 Keto Recipes

In this chapter, we will discuss some delicious keto recipes.

4.1. Muffins of Almond Butter

(Ready in 35 Mins, Serves: 12, Difficulty: Normal)

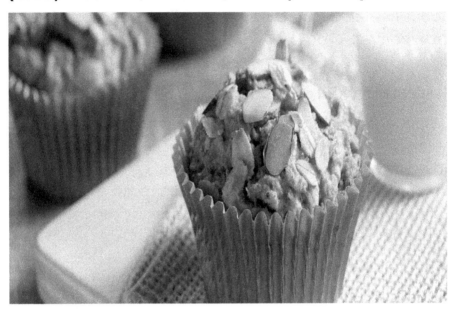

Ingredients:

- Four eggs
- 2 cups almond flour
- 1/4 tsp. salt
- 3/4 cup warm almond butter,
- 3/4 cup almond milk
- 1 cup powdered erythritol
- Two teaspoons baking powder

Instructions:

1. In a muffin cup, put the paper liners before the oven is preheated to 160 degrees Celsius.

2. Mix erythritol, almond meal, baking powder, and salt in a mixing bowl.

3. In another cup, mix the warm almond milk with the almond butter.

4. Drop some ingredients in a dry bowl till they are all combined.

5. In a ready cooker, sprinkle the flour and cook for 22-25 minutes until a clean knife is placed in the center.

6. Cool the bottle for five minutes to cool.

4.2. Breakfast Quesadilla

(Ready in 25 Mins, Serves: 4, Difficulty: Easy)

Ingredients:

- 4 eggs
- 1/4 cup (56 g) salsa
- 1/4 cup (30 g) low-fat Cheddar cheese, shredded
- 8 corn tortillas

Instructions:

1. When it is done, throw in the salsa, and whisk in the cheese to the very top. Sprinkle the oil on a few tortillas and then place a few pieces on an even number of the tortillas' edges.

2. Take the baking sheet. Divide the egg mixture between the tortillas, which is much more challenging. Oil-side up, cover the remaining tortillas. For 3 minutes or before the golden brown heats up, grill the quesadillas on each side. Serve.

4.3. California Breakfast Sandwich

(Ready in 30 Mins, Serves: 6, Difficulty: Easy)

Ingredients:

- 1/2 a cup (90 g) chopped tomato
- 1/2 a cup (60 g) grated Cheddar cheese
- Six whole-wheat English muffins
- 2 ounces (55 g) mushrooms, sliced
- One avocado, sliced
- 6 eggs
- 3/4 cup (120 g) chopped onion
- 1 tbsp. unsalted butter

Instructions:

Beat the eggs together. Brown onion in a large oven-proof or high-sided skillet until clear. It's safe and tidy. Chop up avocado, tomatoes, and champagne onion blend and stir. Blend together. Proofread the attached work. Quickly cook until it's almost cooked. Add the salt, vinegar, and cheese. Spoon with English toasted muffins.

4.4. Stromboli Keto

(Ready in 45 Mins, Serves: 4, Difficulty: Normal)

Ingredients:

- 4 oz. ham
- 4 oz. cheddar cheese
- Salt and pepper
- 4 tbsp. almond flour
- 1¼ cup shredded mozzarella cheese
- 1 tsp. Italian seasoning
- 3 tbsp. coconut flour
- One egg

Instructions:

1. To avoid smoking, stir the mozzarella cheese in the microwave for 1 minute or so.

2. Apply each cup of the melted mozzarella cheese, mix the food, coconut fleece, pepper and salt together. A balanced equilibrium. Then add the eggs and blend again for a while after cooling off.

3. Place the mixture on the parchment pad and place the second layer above it. Through your hands or rolling pin, flatten it into a rectangle.

4. Remove the top sheet of paper and use a butter knife to draw diagonal lines towards the dough's middle. They can be cut one-half of the way on the one side. And cut diagonal points on the other side, too.

5. At the edge of the dough are alternate ham and cheese slices. Then fold on one side, and on the other side, cover the filling.

6. Bake for 15-20 minutes at 226°C; place it on a baking tray.

4.5. Cups of Meat-Lover Pizza

(Ready in 26 Mins, Serves: 12, Difficulty: Easy)

Ingredients:

- 24 pepperoni slices
- 1 cup cooked and crumbled bacon
- 12 tbsp. sugar-free pizza sauce
- 3 cups grated mozzarella cheese
- 12 deli ham slices
- 1 lb. bulk Italian sausage

Instructions

1. Preheat the oven to 375 F Celsius (190 degrees Celsius). Italian brown sausages, soaked in a saucepan of extra fat.

2. Cover the 12-cup ham slices with a muffin tin. Divide it into sausage cups, mozzarella cheese, pizza sauce, and pepperoni slots.

3. Bake for 10 mins at 375. Cook for 1 minute until the cheese pops and the meat tops show on the ends, until juicy.

4. Enjoy the muffin and put the pizza cups to avoid wetting them on paper towels. Uncover or cool down and heat up quickly in the toaster oven or microwave.

4.6. Chicken Keto Sandwich

(Ready in 30 Mins, Serves: 2, Difficulty: Normal)

Ingredients:

For the Bread:

- 3 oz. cream cheese
- ⅛ tsp. cream of tartar Salt
- Garlic powder
- Three eggs

For the Filling:

- 1 tbsp. mayonnaise
- Two slices bacon
- 3 oz. chicken
- 1 tsp. Sriracha
- 2 slices pepper jack cheese
- 2 grape tomatoes
- ¼ avocado

Instructions:

1. Divide the eggs into several cups. Add cream tartar, cinnamon, then beat to steep peaks in the egg whites.

2. In a different bowl, beat the cream cheese. In a white egg mixture, combine the mixture carefully.

3. Place the batter on paper and, like bread pieces, make little square shapes. Gloss over the garlic powder, then bake for 25 mins at 148°C.

4. As the bread bakes, cook the chicken and bacon in a saucepan and season to taste.

5. Remove from the oven and cool when the bread is finished for 10-15 mins. Then add mayo, Sriracha, tomatoes, and mashed avocado, and add fried chicken and bacon to your sandwich.

4.7. Keto Tuna Bites With Avocado

(Ready in 13 Mins, Serves: 8, Difficulty: Very Easy)

Ingredients:

- 10 oz. drained canned tuna
- ⅓ cup almond flour
- ½ cup coconut oil
- ¼ cup mayo
- 1 avocado
- ½ tsp. garlic powder
- ¼ tsp. onion powder
- ¼ cup parmesan cheese
- Salt and pepper

Instructions:

1. Both ingredients are mixed in a dish (excluding cocoa oil). Shape small balls of almond meal and fill them.

2. Fry them with coconut oil (it needs to be hot) in a medium-hot pan until browned on all sides.

4.8. Green Keto Salad

(Ready in 10 Mins, Serves: 1, Difficulty: Easy)

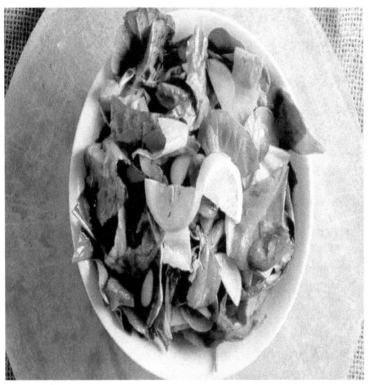

Ingredients:

- 100 g mixed lettuce
- 200 g cucumber
- 2 stalks celery
- 1 tbsp. olive oil
- Salt as per choice
- 1 tsp white wine vinegar or lemon juice

Instructions:

1. With your hands, rinse and cut the lettuce.

2. Cucumber and celery chop.

3. Combine all.

4. For the dressing, add vinegar, salt, and oil.

4.9. Breakfast Enchiladas

(Ready in 1 Hr., Serves: 8, Difficulty: Normal)

Ingredients:

- 12 ounces (340 g) ham, finely chopped
- Eight whole-wheat tortillas
- 4 eggs
- 1 tbsp. flour
- 1/4 tsp. garlic powder
- 1 tsp. Tabasco sauce
- 2 cups (300 g) chopped green bell pepper
- 1 cup (160 g) chopped onion
- 2 1/2 a cup (300 g) grated Cheddar cheese
- 2 cups (475 ml) skim milk
- 1/2 a cup (50 g) chopped scallions

Instructions:

1. Preheat the oven to 350 °F (180 °C). Combine the ham, scallions, bell pepper, tomatoes and cheese. Apply five teaspoons of the mixture to each tortilla and roll-up.

2. In a 30 x 18 x 5-cm (12 x 7 x 2-inch) non-stick pan. In a separate oven, beat together the eggs, milk, garlic, and Tabasco. Cook for 30 minutes with foil, then show the last 10 minutes.

Tip: Serve with a sour cream dollop, salsa, and slices of avocado.

4.10. Keto Mixed Berry Smoothie Recipe

(Ready in 5 Mins, Serves: 4, Difficulty: Easy)

Ingredients:

- 2 scoops Vanilla Collagen
- 1 cup of frozen Mixed Berries
- 2 cups Ice
- 1/4 cup Erythritol Powdered Monk Fruit
- 1 cup Unsweetened Coconut Milk Vanilla

Instructions

1. In a high-speed blender, combine all the ingredients.

2. Use or mix until smooth the "smoothie" setting.

4.11. Low-Carb Tropical Pink Smoothie

(Ready in 5 Mins, Serves: 1, Difficulty: Easy)

Ingredients: (makes 1 smoothie)

- $1/2$ small dragon fruit
- 1 tbsp. chia seeds
- 1 small wedge Gallia, Honeydew
- 1/2 a cup coconut milk *or* heavy whipping cream
- 1 scoop of whey protein powder (vanilla or plain), or gelatin or egg white powder.
- 3-6 drops extract of Stevia *or* other low-carb sweeteners
- 1/2 a cup water
- *Optional:* few ice cubes

Instructions

1. Monitor and place all the components smoothly in a mixer and pulse. Before or after combining this, you can apply the ice.

2. It is possible to include the fruit of a white or pink dragon. Serve.

4.12. Keto Peanut Butter Smoothie

(Ready in 1 Min, Serves: 1, Difficulty: Very Easy)

Ingredients:

- 1/2 a cup almond milk
- 1 tbsp. peanut butter
- 1 tbsp. cocoa powder
- 1-2 tbsp. peanut butter powdered
- 1/4 of avocado
- 1 serving liquid stevia
- 1/4 cup ice

Instructions

1. Add all the ingredients other than the ice and mix well in a food processor.

2. Apply enough milk to the smoothie for the ideal consistency. Add more ice or ground peanut butter to thin it out.

3. Serve it in a glass.

4.13. 5 Minute Keto Cookies & Cream Milkshake

(Ready in 5 Mins, Serves: 2, Difficulty: Easy)

Ingredients:

- $3/4$ cup heavy whipping cream or coconut milk
- Two large squares of grated dark chocolate
- **Optional:** frozen cubes of almond milk/ few ice cubes
- 1 cup unsweetened any nut or almond milk or seed milk
- 1 tsp vanilla powder or vanilla extract sugar-free
- 1-2 tsp Erythritol powdered, few drops of stevia
- $1/3$ cup walnuts or pecans chopped
- 2 tbsp. almond butter, (roasted or sunflower seed)
- 2 tbsp. coconut cream /whipped cream for garnishing

Instructions

1. Place in a blender, mix all the ingredients together (except topping). It is thicker as you blink. The ganache should be lit or topped with other ingredients.

2. Mix the whipped cream into the topping separately. Use 1/2 to 1 cup of milk for pounding. You should have whipped cream in the fridge for three days.

3. Pour some water into a bottle. Drizzle the nuts and butter leftover over the milk.

4.14. Keto Eggnog Smoothie

(Ready in 5 Mins, Serves: 1, Difficulty: Easy)

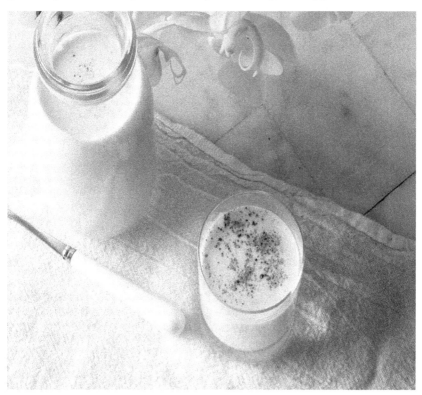

Ingredients:

- 1 Large Egg
- 1 tsp Erythritol
- 1/4 cup whipping cream (coconut cream for dairy-free)
- 1/2 tsp Cinnamon
- 4 Cloves ground approx. ¼ tsp
- 1 tsp Maple Syrup Sugar-Free (optional)

Instructions

In a blender, combine all the ingredients and mix fast for 30 seconds – 1 min.

4.15. Easy Keto Oreo Shake

(Ready in 5 Mins, Serves: 2, Difficulty: Easy)

Ingredients:

- 4 large eggs
- 2 tbsp. black cocoa powder or Dutch-process cocoa powder
- 1 1/2 cups unsweetened cashew milk, almond milk, or water 4 tbsp. roasted almond butter or Keto Butter
- 3 tbsp. Erythritol powdered or Swerve
- 1/4 cup whipping cream
- 1/4 tsp vanilla powder or 1/2 tsp vanilla extract (sugar-free)
- 1/2 a cup whipped cream for garnishing

Instructions

1. Place the frozen or cashew milk/almond milk in an ice cube tray and then freeze them. Under the right conditions (which means don't freeze the shake), miss this step and go on to the next.

2. Stir the cream in a tub of frozen milk. To produce ice cream, add ice cream to the warmed cream. Put some ova somewhere.

3. Apply the soaked nuts, sweetener, cacao powder, and vanilla to the dish. With macadamia, cocoa, cassava, and MCT, these oils are nice to use with MCT oil. Blend until smooth.

6. Apply more whipped cream before serving.

4.16. Keto Eggs Florentine

(Ready in 55 Mins, Serves: 4, Difficulty: Normal)

Ingredients:

- 1 tbsp. of white vinegar
- 1 Cup cleaned, the spinach leaves fresh
- 2 Tablespoons of Parmesan cheese, finely grated
- 2 Chickens
- 2 Eggs
- Ocean salt and chili to compare

Instructions:

1. Boil the spinach in a decent bowl or steam until it waves.

2. Sprinkle with the parmesan cheese to taste.

3. Break and put the bits on a tray. Place the tray on them.

4. Steam a hot water bath, add the vinegar and mix it in a whirlpool with a wooden spoon.

5. Place the egg in the center of the egg, turn the heat over and cover until set (3-4 minutes). Repeat for the second seed.

6. Put the spinach with the egg and drink.

4.17. Loaded Cauliflower (Low Carb, Keto)

(Ready in 20 Mins, Serves: 4, Difficulty: Easy)

Ingredients:

- 1 pound cauliflower
- 3 tablespoons butter
- 4 ounces of sour cream
- 1/4 tsp. garlic powder
- 1 cup cheddar cheese, grated
- 2 slices bacon crumbled and cooked
- 2 tbsp. chives snipped
- pepper and salt to taste

Instructions

1. Chop or dice cauliflower and switch to a microwave-safe oven. Add two water teaspoons and cover with sticking film. Microwave for 5-10 minutes until thoroughly cooked and tender. Empty the excess water, give a minute or two to dry. If you want to strain the cooking water, steam up your cooling flora (or use hot water as normal.)

2. Add the cauliflower to the food processor. Pulse it until smooth and creamy. Mix in the sugar, garlic powder and sour cream. Press it in a cup, then scatter with more cheese, then mix it up. Add pepper and salt.

3. Add the leftover cheese, chives and bacon to the loaded cauliflower. Place the cauliflower under the grill for a few minutes in the microwave to melt the cheese.

4. Serve and enjoy.

4.18. Crispy Drumsticks

(Ready in 1 Hr. 5 Mins, Serves: 4, Difficulty: Normal)

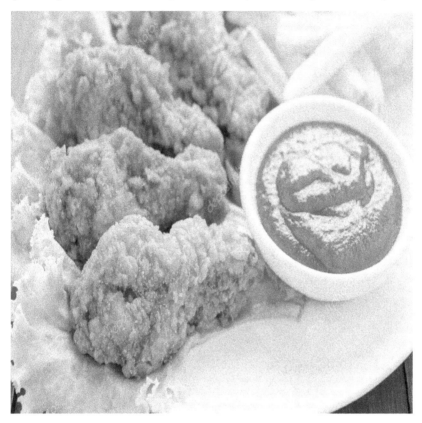

Ingredients:

- Dried thyme
- Olive oil
- 10 – 12 chicken drumsticks (preferably organic)
- Paprika
- Sea salt
- Black pepper

- 4 tbsp. Grass-fed butter or ghee, melted and divided

Instructions

1. Heat the oven to 375 F.

2. Line a rimmed baking sheet.

3. On the parchment paper, in a single sheet of holes between the drumsticks.

4. Mix 1/2 of the melted butter or ghee in olive oil with drumsticks.

5. Sprinkle on thyme and seasoning.

6. Turn it on for 30 minutes. Carefully empty the bottle and switch drumsticks over. When the drumsticks are cooling, produce a thyme and butter mixture again.

7. Return the pie for another 30 minutes (or until finely browned and externally baked).

4.18. Shredded Herbal Cattle

(Ready in 50 Mins, Serves: 4, Difficulty: Normal)

Ingredients:

- 2 tablespoons of rice wine
- 1 tbsp. of olive oil
- 1 pound leg,
- 2 Chipotle peppers in adobo sauce,
- 1 garlic clove chopped,
- Mature tomatoes, peeled and pureed
- 1 yellow onion
- 1/2 tbsp. chopped fresh Mustard
- 1 cup of dried basil
- 1 cup of dried marjoram
- 1/4 cut into strips beef
- 2 medium shaped chipotles crushed
- 1 cup beef bone broth
- Table salt and ground black pepper,
- Parsley, 2 spoonful's of new chives, finely chopped

Instructions:

In an oven, steam the oil in a medium to high heat. Continuously cook beef for six to seven minutes. Add all the ingredients to the beef. Heat and cook for 40 minutes; add the remaining to a moderate-low heat. Then tear the meat, have it.

4.19. Nilaga Filipino Soup

(Ready in 45 Mins, Serves: 4, Difficulty: Normal)

Ingredients:

- 1 Tsp. butter
- 1 tbsp. patis (fish sauce)
- 1 pound of pork ribs, boneless and 1 shallot thinly sliced bits,
- Split 2 garlic cloves, chopped 1 (1/2) "slice of fresh ginger, 1 cup chopped
- 1 cup of fresh tomatoes,
- 1 cup pureed "Corn."
- Cauliflower
- salt and green chili pepper, to taste

Instructions:

1. Melt the butter in a bowl over medium to high heat. Heat the pork ribs for 5-6 minutes on both sides. Stir in the shallot, the garlic and the ginger. Add extra ingredients.

2. Cook, sealed, for 30 to 35 mins. Serve in different containers and remain together.

4.20. Lemon Mahi-Mahi Garlicky

(Ready in 30 Mins, Serves: 4, Difficulty: Normal)

Ingredients:

- Kosher salt
- 4 (4-oz.) mahi-mahi fillets
- Ground black pepper

- 1 lb. asparagus
- 2 tbsp. extra-virgin olive oil,
- 1 lemon
- juice of 1 lemon and zest also
- 3 cloves garlic
- ¼ tsp. of crushed red pepper flakes
- 3 tbsp. butter, divided
- 1 tbsp. freshly parsley chopped, and more for garnish

Instructions:

1. Melt one tbsp. Cook some butter in a large saucepan, then add oil. Season with salt and black pepper. Mahia, add, sauté. Cook for 5 minutes on each side. Transfer to a dish.

2. Apply one tbsp. of oil for the casserole. Cook for 4 minutes and add the spawn. Season with salt and pepper on a pan.

3. Heat butter to the skillet. Add garlic and pepper flakes and simmer until fragrant. Then add lemon zest, juice, and Persil. Break the mahi-mahi into smaller pieces, then add asparagus and sauce.

4. Garnish before consuming.

Conclusions:

An important element to note is eating a great combination of lean meat, greens, and unprocessed carbs. The most efficient way to eat a balanced diet is simply adhering to whole foods, mainly because it is a healthy solution. It is crucial to understand that it is impossible to complete a ketogenic diet.

If you're a woman over 50, you may be far more interested in weight loss. Many women experience decreased metabolism at this age at a rate of about 50 calories per day. It can be incredibly hard to control weight gain by slowing the metabolism combined with less activity, muscle degradation and the potential for greater cravings. Many food options can help women over 50 lose weight and maintain healthy habits, but the keto diet has recently been one of the most popular.

CPSIA information can be obtained
at www.ICGtesting.com
Printed in the USA
BVHW041436070521
606759BV00008B/1489